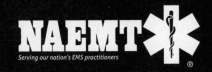

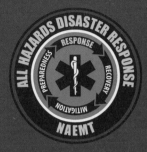

All Hazards Disaster Response

Course Manual

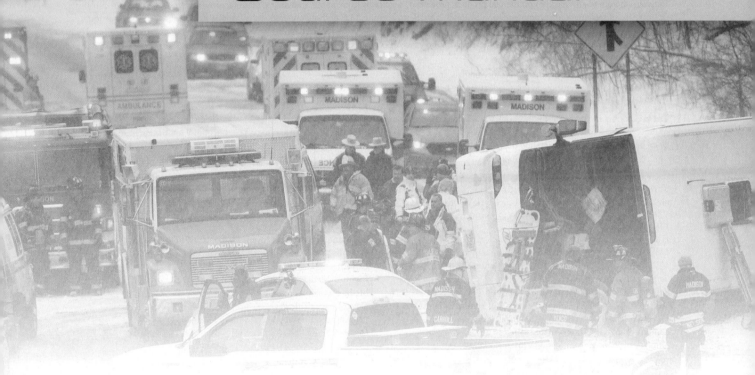

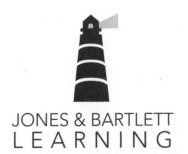

JONES & BARTLETT
LEARNING

World Headquarters
Jones & Bartlett Learning
5 Wall Street
Burlington, MA 01803
978-443-5000
info@jblearning.com
www.jblearning.com

Jones & Bartlett Learning books and products are available through most bookstores and online booksellers. To contact Jones & Bartlett Learning directly, call 800-832-0034, fax 978-443-8000, or visit our website, www.jblearning.com.

Production Credits

General Manager, Safety and Trades: Doug Kaplan
General Manager, Executive Publisher: Kimberly Brophy
VP, Product Development and Executive Editor: Christine Emerton
Senior Acquisitions Editor: Tiffany Sliter
Senior Development Editor: Alison Lozeau
VP, International Sales, Public Safety Group: Matthew Maniscalco
Director of Sales, Public Safety Group: Patricia Einstein
Senior Production Editor: Amanda Clerkin
Director of Marketing Operations: Brian Rooney

VP, Manufacturing and Inventory Control: Therese Connell
Composition: S4Carlisle Publishing Services
Cover Design: Kristin E. Parker
Rights & Media Specialist: Robert Boder
Media Development Editor: Shannon Sheehan
Cover Image (Title Page): © Sean D. Elliot/The Day/AP Photo
Printing and Binding: LSC Communications
Cover Printing: LSC Communications

ISBN: 978-1-284-04104-0

6048

Printed in the United States of America
21 20 19   10 9 8 7 6 5 4 3

CONTENTS

COURSE PLAN

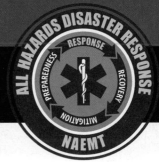

20 minutes	Welcome and Course Introduction
15 minutes	Critical Thinking Skill Station: Hazard Vulnerability Analysis (HVA) Activity
30 minutes	Lesson 1: Structural Fires
30 minutes	Lesson 2: Radiologic Events
20 minutes	Critical Thinking Skill Station: Practitioner Preparedness Self-Assessment
15 minutes	Break
45 minutes	Lesson 3: Natural Disasters and Infrastructure Failures
25 minutes	Lesson 4: Triage
25 minutes	Critical Thinking Skill Station: Triage Simulation Exercise
60 minutes	Lunch
30 minutes	Lesson 5: Transportation Incidents
20 minutes	Critical Thinking Skill Station: LCAN Drill
30 minutes	Lesson 6: Infectious Disease
20 minutes	Critical Thinking Skill Station: Mass-Casualty Tabletop Exercise
15 minutes	Break
30 minutes	Lesson 7: Active Shooter: Evolving Concepts of Care
60 minutes	Critical Thinking Skill Station: Active Shooter Tabletop Exercise
50 minutes	Post-Assessment

Welcome and Introduction

Catastrophes and disasters are becoming more of a common occurrence every year. The number of windstorm-related disasters (wildfires, severe thunderstorms, and derechos) is trending upward since 2006. Losses from hurricanes and flooding have tripled since the year 2000. How well prepared are we?

The National Association of EMTs (NAEMT) surveyed its members about their training for disaster response and found that most agencies do not require training, yet a disaster can occur in any jurisdiction (**FIGURE 1**).

The American College of Emergency Physicians (ACEP) developed a program on all hazards disaster response designed to prepare prehospital providers with the knowledge and skills to care for patients and function during the initial aftermath of a disaster or mass-casualty event. The NAEMT assembled the following team of subject-matter experts to develop a course for this program.

Course Authors:

- Faizan H. Arshad, MD (lead author)
- Sean J. Britton, MPA, NRP, CEM
- Bradford Newbury, MPA, NRP, I/C

Course Medical Director:

- Craig Manifold, DO, FACEP, FAAEM, FAEMS

Course Contributors:

- Michael J. Ward, MGA
- Bill McDonald, PhD, FACEM, NRP
- Leslie Hernandez, EdD, NRP, FP-C
- Ray Casillas, Fire Fighter/Sr. Swat Paramedic

All Hazards Disaster Response (AHDR) focuses on the basic principles and key components of disaster management. Content is organized around the phases of emergency management—mitigation, preparedness, response, and recovery. Broad content categories cover the principal knowledge and skills required for an effective all hazards disaster response by prehospital practitioners at all levels (**FIGURE 2**).

This course is scenario-based. Realistic scenarios cover a variety of potential events, including notice and nonnotice, natural, and human-made events. All phases—mitigation, preparedness, response, and recovery—are covered in the scenarios. However, the course focuses on response, emphasizes a team approach, and weaves in public health

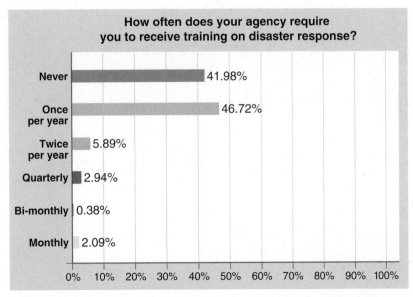

Figure 1 Disaster response training.

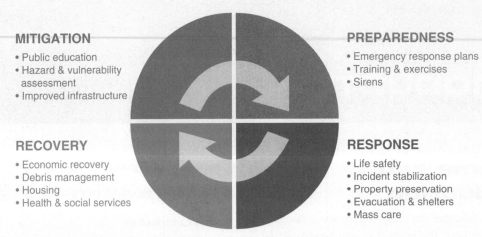

Figure 2 Systems-based approach to disasters.

roles, tasks, and language. Coordinated planning and recovery are integrated into each scenario. Blended learning strategies include interactive presentation as well as leader-led and self-study sessions. Instructors and learners are encouraged to learn more about the topics discussed by exploring the print and online resources provided at the end of each chapter.

This course manual is a required component for the AHDR program and provides an important reference for the AHDR components covered in the course.

Structural Fires

OBJECTIVES

After studying this chapter, you will be able to:

- Identify three key questions regarding resource management.

- Describe patient management objectives when resources are limited.

- Apply care principles of managing patients during different types of patient presentations typical of disaster response.

- Describe strategies for allocating limited resources to optimize patient outcomes during triage and treatment.

- Identify the key decision drivers in changing the patient care focus from individual outcomes to population outcomes.

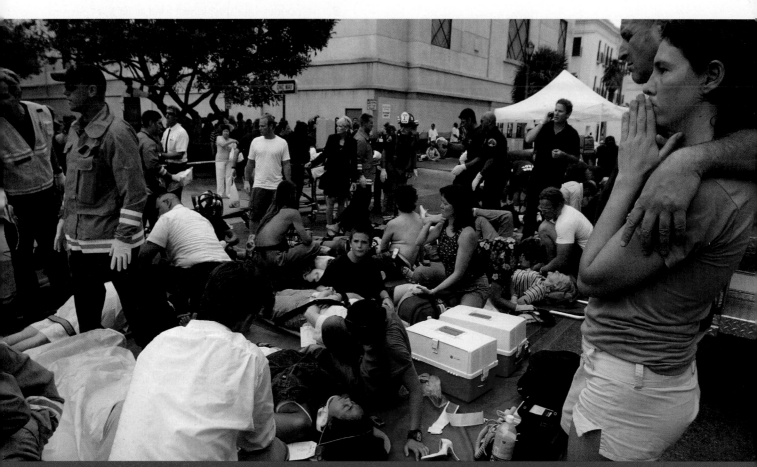

EMS Response Within the Incident Command System

A structure fire involving injuries presents a dynamic event requiring prehospital providers to determine the magnitude of the need and set out the emergency medical services (EMS) incident command framework to provide the best patient care with the available resources.

The first arriving EMS providers must take the time to perform an overall scene assessment. The goals of this assessment are to evaluate any potential hazards, estimate the potential number of casualties, determine what additional medical resources will be needed at the scene, and evaluate whether any specialized equipment or personnel are needed. This assessment is done with the assistance of the **incident commander (IC)**, who is the person responsible for all aspects of a response to an incident. The IC manages all incident operations, sets priorities, and develops an **incident action plan (IAP)**. The IAP is a continuously updated outline of the overall strategy, tactics, and risk management plans to respond to and mitigate the effects of the event.

incident commander (IC) The person responsible for all aspects of a response to an incident, including developing incident objectives, managing all incident operations, setting priorities, and defining the incident command system for the specific response; the IC position must always be filled.

incident action plan (IAP) A continuously updated outline of the overall strategy, tactics, and risk management plans developed by the incident commander.

incident command system (ICS) An emergency response system that defines the roles and responsibilities to be assumed by personnel and the operating procedures to be used in the management and direction of emergency operations.

National Incident Management System (NIMS) A plan that provides a consistent nationwide template to enable federal, state, tribal, and local governments; the private sector; and nongovernmental organizations to work together to prepare for, prevent, respond to, recover from, and mitigate the effects of incidents, regardless of cause, size, location, or complexity, so as to reduce the loss of life, damage to property, and harm to the environment.

The **incident command system (ICS)** is part of the **National Incident Management System (NIMS)** Command and Management component. Local emergency response agencies are required to adopt ICS to remain eligible for federal disaster assistance. Adopting this system requires training in the core NIMS curriculum (listed in order of typical completion):

- IS 700: National Incident Management System (NIMS), an Introduction
- ICS 100: Introduction to the Incident Command System
- ICS 200: ICS for Single Resources and Initial Action Incidents
- IS 800: National Response Framework, an Introduction
- Appropriate position-specific training

CHECK YOUR KNOWLEDGE

The individual responsible for all aspects of managing an emergency incident is the:

A. first arriving command-qualified responder.
B. responder with the highest level of NIMS credentials.
C. incident commander.
D. chief administrative officer of the jurisdiction.

The EMS Branch

An apartment fire with 20 injured occupants represents a major event in which the IC will expect the first arriving prehospital care providers to establish the medical branch under the ICS. Under the medical branch director, there are up to nine tasks that may require a group supervisor or unit leader:

1. Triage
2. Treatment
3. Transportation
4. Communications
5. Extrication
6. Medical staging
7. Supply
8. Landing zone
9. Reconnaissance (usually referred to simply as *recon*)

For this scenario, the first arriving ambulance crew established the medical branch director and triage unit leader. As the second arriving ambulance, your crew is directed to establish the triage unit (**FIGURE 1-1**).

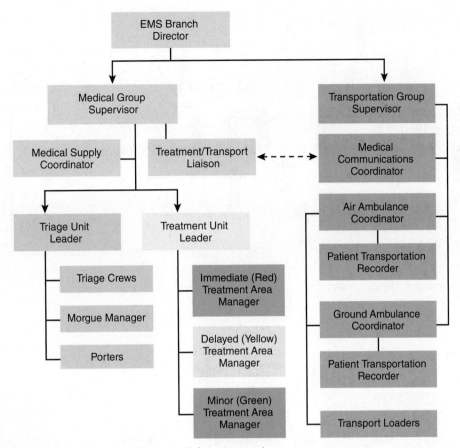

Figure 1-1 EMS branch command positions and the triage unit.

Reproduced from Northern Virginia EMS Operations Board (May 2013) *EMS Multiple Casualty Incident Manual* (2nd ed.). Fairfax, VA: Northern Virginia Emergency Response System. Accessed at https://www.nvers.org/fireems/fireems-documents/nova-procedural-and-training-packages/ on December 21, 2016.

Setting Up the Transportation Group

As the second ambulance arriving at the apartment fire, you are directed to establish the transportation group. The transportation group manages patient movement and accountability from the scene to receiving hospitals or alternative care sites. The transportation group supervisor works with the treatment group supervisor to establish adequately sized, easily identifiable patient loading areas; designates an ambulance staging area; and maintains communication with the medical group supervisor for situation briefings and resource allocation.

For our apartment fire event, there can be one **patient intake point (PIP)**. The PIP is the physical location prior to entering the treatment areas through which all patients are funneled and where a disaster tag is applied. When possible, the disaster tag should be scanned into the patient tracking system. There is also one **patient exit point (PEP)**. The PEP is the physical location through which the patient exits the scene via the transport unit (air or ground); it is here that the transport stub is collected (by the transport recorder)

from the disaster tag and affixed to the transport record. If available, the departure should be scanned into the patient tracking system. **FIGURE 1-2** shows how the medical branch can be laid out.

patient intake point (PIP) The physical location prior to entering the treatment areas through which all patients are funneled and where a disaster tag is applied. When possible, the disaster tag should be scanned into the patient tracking system.

patient exit point (PEP) The physical location through which the patient exits the scene via the transport unit (air or ground); it is here that the transport stub is collected (by the transport recorder) from the disaster tag and affixed to the transport record. If available, the departure should be scanned into the patient tracking system.

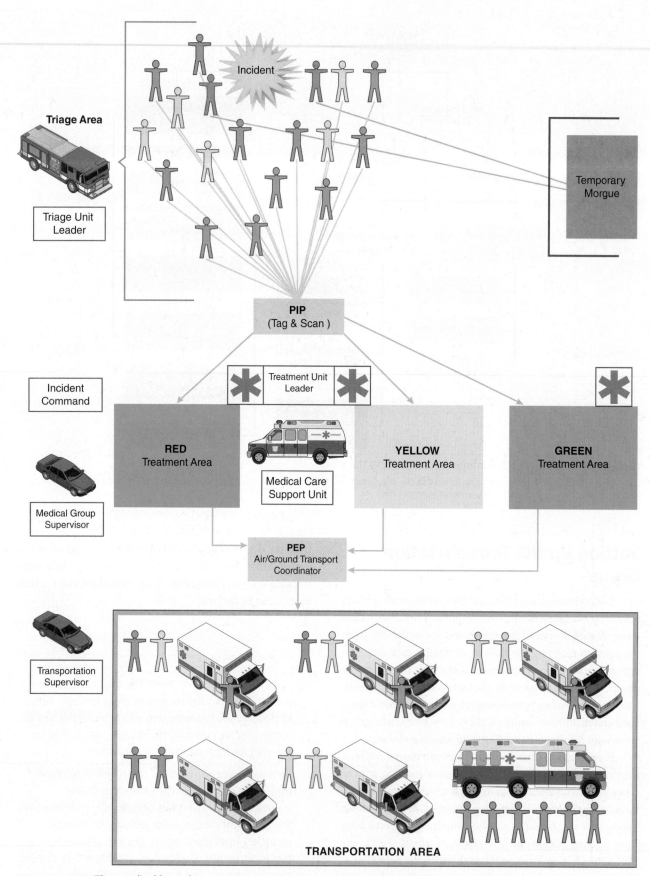

Figure 1-2 The medical branch.

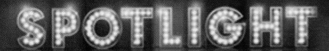

Transport Group Supervisor Duty Checklist

- Obtain a situation briefing from the medical branch director and secure radio channel for transport group operations.
- Establish a log to document the destination of each patient and which unit transported the patient.
- Ensure that enough transport units are called to handle the patient count. Plan on sending two intermediate patients per ambulance, adding delayed or minor patients as space permits.

- Determine destination hospitals to distribute patients to as many appropriate hospitals as practical.
- Coordinate with EMS dispatch whether transport units should return to the incident or clear the incident after delivering the patient to the hospital.
- Appoint and brief a ground ambulance coordinator and assistants.
- If available, don a command position vest.
- Consider a one-way traffic pattern to facilitate access to

and egress from the patient loading area.
- Ensure that enough responders are available to promptly load patients into ambulances.
- Coordinate with the air ambulance coordinator for any medivac transports.
- Advise the medical branch director of additional resource needs.
- Forward all logs, records, and checklists to the medical branch director when demobilizing a transportation group.

 CHECK YOUR KNOWLEDGE

The medical branch director position within the ICS is:

A. required to be a paramedic.
B. established by the first arriving EMS unit to the incident.
C. predesignated by the operational medical director.
D. required to have completed ICS 240A, Leadership and Influence.

Crisis Standards of Care

Assessing, treating, and transporting 20 people injured at a structure fire would overwhelm the medical resources in many communities. Catastrophic disasters throughout the world compelled the Department of Health and Human Services to ask the Institute of Medicine (now called the National Academy of Medicine) to convene a committee of experts to develop national guidance for use by state and local public health officials and health-sector agencies and institutions in establishing and implementing standards of care that should apply in disaster situations—both naturally occurring and human-made—under

conditions of scarce resources. In 2009, the Committee on Guidance for Establishing Standards of Care for Use in Disaster Situations defined these "crisis standards of care" (CSCs) to be a

substantial change in the usual health care operations and the level of care it is possible to deliver . . . justified by specific circumstances and . . . formally declared by a state government in recognition that crisis operations will be in effect for a sustained period.

Professional care delivered in a catastrophic disaster may need to be modified to address the demands of the situation, including focusing more intently on the needs of the entire affected community. **TABLE 1-1** differentiates activities under conventional, contingency, and crisis conditions.

 CHECK YOUR KNOWLEDGE

Under what conditions would an EMS agency not attempt to resuscitate a patient in unwitnessed cardiac arrest that is not ventricular fibrillation?

A. Crisis conditions
B. Contingency conditions
C. Conventional conditions
D. Under no conditions

TABLE 1-1 Potential EMS Response Adaptations Under Conventional, Contingency, and Crisis Conditions[a]

	Conventional	Contingency	Crisis[b]
Dispatch	• Consider initial autoanswer during times of high call volume for medical emergencies	• Prioritize calls according to potential threat to life; "pend" apparently non-life-threatening calls (note this requires a medically trained dispatcher, not available at many public safety answering points [PSAPs])	• Decline response to calls without evident potential threat to life (also requires a medically trained dispatcher)
Response	• Modify resource assignments (e.g., only fire/rescue dispatched to motor vehicle crashes unless EMS are clearly required, single-agency EMS responses if fire agencies are overtaxed) • Seek mutual-aid assistance from surrounding areas	• Modify resource assignments to a greater extent • Change EMS assignments to closest available unit rather than advanced life support (ALS)/basic life support (BLS) • Consider staffing configuration changes (e.g., from two paramedics to one paramedic plus one emergency medical technician [EMT]-B) • Consider requests for disaster assistance	• Request EMS units from emergency management (if possible) • Consider use of National Guard ambulances or other assets • Utilize scheduled BLS providers to answer emergency calls • Change staffing to one medical provider, one driver • Further modify resource assignments as possible • Attempt no resuscitation of cardiac arrests (except ventricular fibrillation [VF] witnessed by EMS)
Patient assessment	• Allow patients with very minor injuries to use their own transportation	• Encourage patients with minor injury/illness to use their own transportation	• Assess patients and decline to transport those without significant injury/illness (according to guidance from EMS medical director)
Transportation	• Transport patients to the closest appropriate facility (rather than the facility of the patient's choice)	• Consider batched transports—answer subsequent call(s) before transporting stable patients to the hospital	• Decline transports as above; employ batch transports as needed

[a] EMS volumes will fluctuate significantly over time; thus, conventional, contingency, and crisis conditions may all occur in a single operational period. Dispatchers must therefore have excellent situational awareness of resources and deployment of personnel to provide the best service possible at a given time and have practice in managing these scenarios.

[b] Crisis adaptations often require state or at least city declarations of emergency, as well as relief from usual staffing and response requirements of the state (often through a governor's emergency order).

Patient Management

Trauma patients die from massive acute blood loss, severe injury to vital organs, and airway obstruction or ventilator failure. At the cellular level, these patients are dying from shock, the failure of energy production within the body. Prehospital trauma life support is designed to reverse the shock process through appropriate interventions aimed at improving oxygenation and controlling hemorrhage during the golden period to prevent the onset of irreversible shock.

Burned Patients

EMS providers see burns as horrifying and frightening events. During the initial event size-up, prehospital care providers must gather as much information about the burning substance as possible and must determine whether the substance contains hazardous materials. This information is important both for the safety of responders and for development of a patient care plan.

The most common cause of death for a fire victim is not from the direct complications of the burn wound, but from complications of respiratory failure. Inhalation of toxic fumes from smoke is a greater predictor of burn mortality than is the age of the patient or the size of the burn. Because life-threatening complications from smoke inhalation may not manifest for several days, prehospital care providers need to consider carbon monoxide or hydrogen cyanide poisoning in their patient assessment.

Thermal Burn Injuries

A major consideration when managing thermal burn injuries is the body surface area (BSA) involved. Skin is crucial in maintaining body temperature and preventing the loss of water. **FIGURE 1-3** shows the Lund-Browder chart, which allows providers to map out the burned areas and then determine the size of the burn based on the reference table.

Life-threatening thermal burn injuries involve insult to multiple systems. Heat from the fire can cause edema of the airway above the vocal cords. Thermal burn patients continue to deteriorate over time, and providers need to be vigilant to maintain a patent airway and watch for narrowing of the airway due to edema.

The depth of a burn also continues after treatment begins, with the final determination of the depth of the burn calculated up to 48 hours after the injury. Circumferential burns of the trunk or limbs can produce a life- or limb-threatening condition from the thick, inelastic eschar that is formed. Circumferential burns of the chest can constrict the chest wall to such a degree that the patient is unable to inhale and suffocates. Circumferential burns of the extremities can create a tourniquet-like effect that can render an arm or leg pulseless. Therefore, all circumferential burns should be handled as an emergency, and patients should be transported to a burn center or, if a burn center is not available, to the local trauma center.

Burn patients are trauma patients and may have sustained injuries other than thermal injuries. Burns are obvious and

Region	%
Head	
Neck	
Ant. Trunk	
Post. Trunk	
Right arm	
Left arm	
Buttocks	
Genitalia	
Right leg	
Left leg	
Total burn	

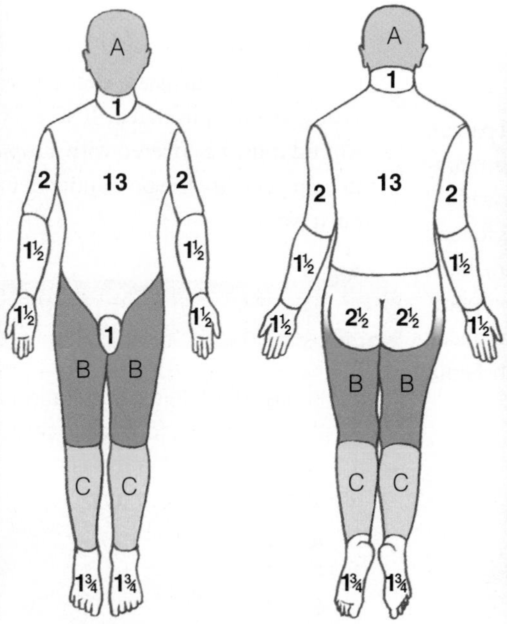

Relative percentages of body surface area affected by growth

Age (years)	A (½ of head)	B (½ of one thigh)	C (½ of one leg)
0	9½	2¾	2½
1	8½	3¼	2½
5	6½	4	2¾
10	5½	4¼	3
15	4½	4½	3¼
Adult	3½	4¾	3

Figure 1-3 Lund-Browder chart.

Data from Lund, C. C., and Browder, N. C. *Surg. Gynecol. Obstet.* 1944. 79: 352–358.

sometimes intimidating injuries, but it is vital to assess for other, less obvious internal injuries that may be more immediately life threatening than the burns. For our apartment fire example, patients may leap from windows or elements of the structure may have fallen on them. In such instances, the patient will have sustained both burns and associated trauma. The immediate life threat is hemorrhage from the traumatic injury, not the burn.

Fluid Resuscitation

Large amounts of IV fluids must be administered over the course of the first day postburn to prevent a burn patient from going into hypovolemic shock. This fluid resuscitation begins in the prehospital setting. Burn patients lose a substantial amount of intravascular fluid owing to obligatory whole body edema and evaporative losses at the site of the burn. The challenge is to maintain an effective level of fluid resuscitation to treat the patient without producing complications. Inadequate administration of IV fluids may lead to hypovolemia and cardiovascular collapse.

Fluid resuscitation is achieved by administering Ringer's lactate or other balanced saline solution. Providers calculate the amount by using the **Consensus formula**:

4 mL × kg body weight × % total body surface area (TBSA) burned (second degree and higher)

Half of that amount will be administered in the first 8 hours after the time of the injury. The rest will be infused over the next 16 hours.

Prehospital Management of Critically Burned Patients

The continuing prehospital care of a critically burned patient involves decreasing the chance of further tissue damage, maintaining a patent airway, providing pain control, and providing fluid resuscitation. Prehospital providers must reassess for any trauma or preexisting medical conditions that may have been missed during the initial care. They should consider complications of carbon monoxide and cyanide poisoning and evaluate the administration of a cyanide antidote or hydroxocobalamin if allowed by local protocol.

Consensus formula A formula used to calculate a range for resuscitative-phase fluid replacement (lactated Ringer's solution) in the first 24 hours when the fluid shifts and the risk for hypovolemic shock is the greatest.

Transport or Transfer to a Burn Center

The following types of burns should be referred to a qualified burn center (i.e., one approved by the American Burn Association):

- Partial-thickness burns greater than 10% TBSA
- Burns that involve the face, hands, feet, genitalia, perineum, or major joints
- Third-degree burns in any age group
- Electrical burns, including lightning injury
- Chemical burns
- Inhalation injury
- Burn injury in patients with preexisting medical disorders that could complicate management, prolong recovery, or affect mortality
- Any patients with burns and concomitant trauma (such as fractures) in which the burn injury poses the greater risk of morbidity or mortality
  - If the trauma poses the greater immediate risk, the patient initially may be stabilized in a trauma center before being transferred to a burn unit.
  - Physician judgment is necessary in such situations and should be in concert with the regional medical control plan and triage protocols.
- Burn injury in children if the nearest hospitals do not have qualified personnel or equipment for the care of children
- Burn injury in patients who will require special social, emotional, or long-term rehabilitative intervention

Within hours of arrival at a burn center, simple debridement of the wound is undertaken. This process may simply involve removal of devitalized tissue. In some burn centers full-thickness burns are excised soon after admission and skin grafting is initiated. If surgery is not performed, the wound must be covered with a topical antimicrobial agent to help decrease the possibility of bacterial infection of the burn wound.

 CHECK YOUR KNOWLEDGE

In providing fluid resuscitation for a burn patient, the Consensus formula is calculated to provide half of the fluid in the first _____ hours after time of the injury.

A. 4
B. 6
C. 8
D. 12

Spontaneous Volunteers

When disaster—natural or human-made—strikes a community, specific emergency management and nonprofit organizations respond according to a preestablished plan. Each of these designated organizations has a specific role to play in ensuring an effective response to and recovery from the disaster's devastation. Yet one element within the present system continues to pose a challenge: spontaneous, unaffiliated volunteers.

Spontaneous, unaffiliated volunteers—our neighbors and ordinary citizens—often arrive on-site at a disaster ready to help. However, because they are not associated with any part of the existing emergency management response system, their offers of help are often underutilized and even problematic to professional responders.

Credentialing Spontaneous Volunteers

These volunteers may not have the training or experience necessary for the response efforts or they may be skilled individuals, as in former or current military personnel, off-duty responders, nurses, or physicians. It is important to have a plan for credentialing or identifying volunteers. At the Boston Marathon bombings, no tracking of volunteers took place and no post-bloodborne exposure was tracked or identified.

Credentialing ensures and validates the identity and attributes (e.g., affiliations, skills, or privileges) of professionals or members of response teams through established standards, allowing a community to plan for, request, and have confidence in resources deployed from other jurisdictions for emergency assistance. Credentialing also ensures that personnel resources match requests and supports effective management of deployed responders.

> ✔ **CHECK YOUR KNOWLEDGE**
>
> Advantages of credentialing spontaneous volunteers include:
>
> **A.** identification of volunteers' skills or credentials.
> **B.** documentation of volunteer contact information for bloodborne exposure follow-up.
> **C.** effective management of deployed volunteer responders.
> **D.** All of the above

Surge Capacity

Surge capacity is the ability to evaluate and care for a markedly increased volume of patients that challenges or exceeds normal operating capacity. As introduced in the Crisis Standards of Care section, surge capacity is divided into three segments: conventional, contingency, and crisis.

Four Components of Surge Capacity

Surge capacity comprises the following four components:

1. **Staff.** Personnel
2. **Stuff.** Supplies and equipment
3. **Structure.** Facility
4. **Systems.** Integrated management policies and procedures

FIGURE 1-4 describes the relationship of these four components.

The American College of Emergency Physicians Position on Surge Capacity

The American College of Emergency Physicians defines surge capacity as follows:

> Surge capacity is a measurable representation of ability to manage a sudden influx of patients. It is dependent on a well-functioning incident management system and the variables of space, supplies, staff, and any special considerations (contaminated or contagious patients, for example).

Health care systems must develop and maintain outpatient and inpatient surge capacity for the triage, treatment, and tracking of patients at the facility or in alternative sites of care or alternative hospitals during infectious disease outbreaks, hazardous materials exposures, and mass-casualty incidents (MCIs). Health care facility and system plans should maximize conventional capacity, as well as plan for contingency capacity (adapting patient care spaces to provide functionally equivalent care) and crisis capacity (adapting to the level of care provided to the resources available when usual care is impossible).

> **surge capacity** The ability to evaluate and care for a markedly increased volume of patients that challenges or exceeds normal operating capacity.

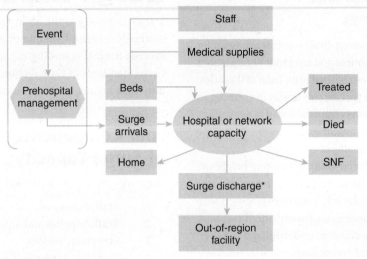

Determinants of Surge Capacity

Figure 1-4 The determinants of surge capacity.

*Note: I am Indebted to Sam Benson, EMT-P, New York City Office of Emergency Management
for the notion of "surge discharge."   —N. Hupert, M.D., M.P.H.

© Jones & Bartlett Learning.

Development of surge capacity requires augmenting existing capacity. It also involves creating capacity by limiting elective appointments and procedures, and practicing "surge discharge" of patients who can be effectively managed in nonhospital environments. Effective surge capacity planning integrates facility plans with a regional disaster response program involving other area health care institutions and considers hazard vulnerability assessments and historical natural disaster threats.

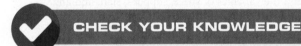

CHECK YOUR KNOWLEDGE

When confronting a sudden influx of patients, EMS providers may be required to:

A. expand their scope of care.
B. transport patients to alternative sites for care.
C. withhold ALS treatment in the field.
D. rely on standing orders in place of on-line medical control.

Multiple Fatalities

A mass-fatality incident (MFI) is a situation in which more fatal accidents occur than can be managed by local resources. MFIs may be human-made, such as hazardous materials releases, transportation accidents, or terrorist attacks, or they may be the result of natural disasters, such as earthquakes, floods, or severe weather. However, when a gunman kills five people, it would probably be considered an MCI and not an MFI if it occurs in a major city.

Family and friends of loved ones may come to the scene. You must be prepared to have the scene secured by law enforcement and shield the bodies from view of the public and media. Where would you get body bags, and how many does your local community have access to? Where could you get an additional supply if needed?

Recovery of the deceased is the first stage in the identification process. There will be tremendous pressure from surviving family members, public officials, the media, and others to rapidly recover and identify the deceased following an MFI. EMS providers must be aware of the tasks associated with forensic body recovery.

Clinical Issues

The scene of the MFI may be a crime scene, in which case the bodies would have to be cleared by law enforcement prior to moving them. Dead bodies do not cause epidemics or pose public health risks, as usually occurs after natural disasters. The risk to the public is negligible if they do not touch dead bodies. The surviving population is much more likely to spread disease than are the dead bodies.

There is the potential (but as yet undocumented) risk of contamination of drinking water supplies by fecal material released from dead bodies. Most disaster-related fatalities are the result of some traumatic mechanism of injury, not disease. Most disaster victims are not likely to be sick with epidemic-causing infections (i.e., Ebola, cholera, typhoid, and anthrax). However, those that are must be handled with appropriate infection control procedures. Some victims will have chronic blood infections (hepatitis and HIV), tuberculosis, or diarrheal disease. Most infectious organisms do not survive beyond 48 hours in a dead body. An exception is HIV, which has been found 6 days postmortem. The Ebola and Marburg viruses have been known to survive up to 5 days on contaminated surfaces.

EMS providers handling human remains have a small risk through contact with blood and feces (bodies often leak feces after death) of being affected by hepatitis B and C, HIV, tuberculosis, and diarrheal disease. Workers should also be cognizant of the hazards posed by highly fragmented remains; for example, body fluids may be dripping from trees (e.g., airline disaster), may be soaked into surrounding soil, or may become an inhalation hazard with airborne dust in collapsed buildings.

Although not immediately relevant to EMS response to an MFI, a key to general safety in the handling of dead bodies is ensuring safe cultural practices and education of the community. As seen in the 2014 West African Ebola outbreak, cultural practices combined with poor understanding of viral transmission greatly exacerbated the propagation of the disease through direct contact with infected corpses.

CHECK YOUR KNOWLEDGE

When assisting at an MFI, EMS providers need to:

A. use standard infection control procedures.
B. wear Level C chemical protective clothing with respirator.
C. wear Level B chemical protective clothing with filter mask.
D. use self-contained breathing apparatus.

Fire Fighter Rehabilitation

Rehabilitation is an intervention designed to mitigate the effects of physical, physiological, and emotional stress of firefighting in order to sustain a fire fighter's ability to work, improve performance, and decrease the likelihood of on-scene injury or death. Studies have shown that most fire fighter injuries and deaths occur during the various active phases of fire suppression. Many of these deaths and injuries can be prevented through use of the rehabilitation process. Key objectives of rehabilitation include the following:

- Relief from climate and environmental conditions
- Rest and recovery
- Active cooling or heating
- Rehydration
- Calorie and electrolyte replacement
- Medical monitoring
- Member accountability
- Release from the rehabilitation process

In the following circumstances, the company or crew must enter a formal rehabilitation area, receive a medical evaluation, and rest with hydration for a minimum of 20 minutes:

- Following the depletion of two 30-minute self-contained breathing apparatus (SCBA) cylinders
- Following the depletion of one 45- or 60-minute SCBA cylinder
- Whenever encapsulating chemical protective clothing is worn
- Following 40 minutes of intense work without a SCBA

The guidelines are based on SCBA use because this is the easiest thing for fire fighters to remember. They almost always know how many SCBA cylinders they have expended. Time tends to compress for those who are involved in emergency operations, and fire fighters often lose track of time. It may be necessary to designate someone as a time recorder during the incident to ensure that crews are rotating out as necessary.

Criteria for Further Medical Evaluation

Each fire department needs to establish criteria in their standard operating procedures regarding vital signs that require medical treatment. In general, the following criteria may be used, unless locally validated criteria are established:

- Pulse in excess of 120 bpm
- Body temperature in excess of 100.5°F (38°C)
- Diastolic blood pressure above 90 mm Hg
- Systolic blood pressure above 130 mm Hg

In addition to simply taking vital signs, rehabilitation personnel should look for other possible clues of injury or distress, including chest pain, shortness of breath, altered level of consciousness, extreme fatigue, poor skin color, and similar symptoms. Any members who have unacceptable vital signs or who exhibit any other signs of an injury or illness should be sent to the medical evaluation or treatment unit for further evaluation and treatment.

 CHECK YOUR KNOWLEDGE

Clinical criteria for further medical evaluation of fire fighters while in rehabilitation include:

A. weight loss since start of work shift.
B. body temperature.
C. pH blood level.
D. urine color.

SUMMARY

- A structure fire involving injuries presents a dynamic event requiring prehospital providers to determine the magnitude of the need and set out the emergency medical services (EMS) incident command framework to provide the best patient care with the available resources.
- The first arriving ambulance crew at a scene establishes the medical branch director and triage unit leader. The second arriving ambulance crew reports to the incident commander for assignment.
- Catastrophic disasters throughout the world compelled the Department of Health and Human Services to ask the Institute of Medicine to convene a committee of experts to develop national guidance for use by state and local public health officials and health-sector agencies and institutions in establishing and implementing standards of care that should apply in disaster situations—both naturally occurring and human-made—under conditions of scarce resources.
- Trauma patients die from massive acute blood loss, severe injury to vital organs, and airway obstruction or ventilator failure. Prehospital trauma life support is designed to reverse the shock process through appropriate interventions aimed at improving oxygenation and controlling hemorrhage during the golden period.
- When disaster—natural or human-made—strikes a community, specific emergency management and nonprofit organizations respond according to a preestablished plan. Spontaneous, unaffiliated volunteers often arrive on-site at a disaster ready to help.
- Surge capacity is the ability to evaluate and care for an increased volume of patients that challenges or exceeds normal operating capacity. Surge capacity is divided into three segments: conventional, contingency, and crisis.
- A mass-fatality incident (MFI) is a situation in which more fatal accidents occur than can be managed by local resources. An MFI may be either human-made or the result of natural disasters.
- Fire fighter rehabilitation is an intervention designed to mitigate the effects of physical, physiological, and emotional stress of firefighting in order to sustain a fire fighter's ability to work, improve performance, and decrease the likelihood of on-scene injury or death.

REFERENCES AND ADDITIONAL RESOURCES

Aehlert, B. (Ed.). (2011). *Paramedic practice today: Above and beyond* (revised reprint). Burlington, MA: Jones and Bartlett.

Altevogt, B. M., Stroud, C., Hanson, S. L., Hanfling, D., and Gostin, L. O. (Eds.). (2009). *Committee on guidance for establishing standards of care for use in disaster situations*. Institute of Medicine. National Academy of Sciences. National Academies Press. Retrieved from http://www.ct.gov/dph/lib/dph/legal/soc/iom_crisis _standard_letter_report.pdf

Committee on Trauma. (2006). *Guidelines for the operations of burn units: Resources for optimal care of the injured patient* (pp. 79–86). Chicago, IL: American College of Surgeons.

Cordner, S., Coninx, R., Kim, H.-J., van Alphen, D., and Tidball-Binz, M. (2016). *Management of dead bodies: A field manual for first responders* (2nd ed). Washington, DC: Pan American Health Organization.

Federal Emergency Management Agency. (2011). *National Incident Management System: Training program*. Washington, DC: U.S. Department of Homeland Security.

Federal Emergency Management Agency. (2012, June). *Operational templates and guidance for EMS mass incident deployment*. Department of Homeland Security. Retrieved from https://www.usfa.fema.gov /downloads/pdf/publications/templates_guidance_ems_mass_incident_deployment.pdf

Federal Emergency Management Agency. (2013). *National response framework* (2nd ed.). Washington, DC: U.S. Department of Homeland Security.

Hanfling, D., Altevogt, B. M., Viswanathan, K., and Gostin, L. O. (Eds.). (2012). *Crisis standards of care: A systems framework for catastrophic disaster response. Volume 1: Introduction and CSC framework*. Washington, DC: Institute of Medicine of the National Academies.

Los Angeles County Emergency Medical Services Agency. (2013, January 31). *Mass fatality guide for healthcare entities*. Los Angeles, CA: Los Angeles County Department of Health Services.

Northern Virginia EMS Operations Board. (2013, May). *EMS multiple casualty incident manual* (2nd ed.). Fairfax, VA: Northern Virginia Emergency Response System. Retrieved from https://www.nvers.org/fireems /fireems-documents/nova-procedural-and-training-packages/

UPS Foundation. (n.d.). *Managing spontaneous volunteers in times of disaster: The synergy of structure and good intention*. Washington, DC: Points of Light Foundation and Volunteer Center National Network. Retrieved from https://www.fema.gov/pdf/donations/ManagingSpontaneousVolunteers.pdf

U.S. Fire Administration. (2008, February). *Emergency incident rehabilitation*. Washington, DC: Federal Emergency Management Agency.

CHAPTER

2 Radiologic Events

OBJECTIVES

After studying this chapter, you will be able to:

- Gain familiarity with operational response to a radiologic incident.

- Gain appreciation for the priorities and goals of incident command during a radiologic event.

- Differentiate between a radiologic dispersion device (RDD), radiologic exposure device (RED), radiologic

incendiary device (RID), and improvised nuclear device (IND).

- Know the limits of safe operating times based on radiation dose.

- Learn the effective use of current radiation detection devices and their functional limits.

- Develop a broad understanding of the special clinical considerations during a radiologic event.

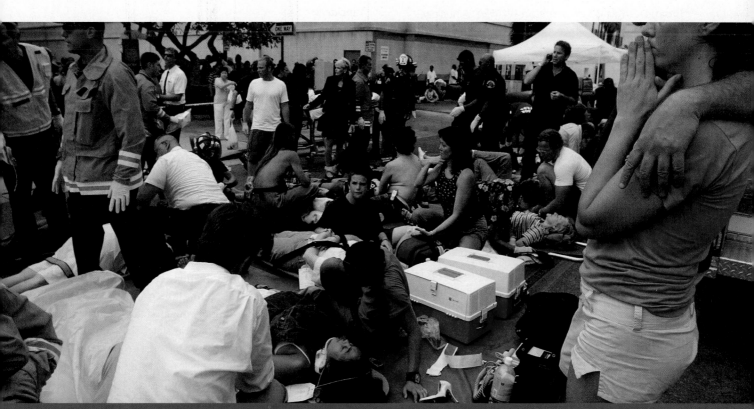

When Does a Radiologic Event Become a Disaster?

Even though the nature of radiologic hazards has not changed in more than six decades, there is something about radiation that spooks us. The term *dirty bombs* has a sinister sound, but of all the terrorist CBRN (chemical, biologic, radiologic, nuclear) threats, radiologic events using a radiologic dispersion device (RDD) are certainly not weapon of mass destruction (WMD) events. The military defines WMD as a nuclear, biologic, or chemical weapon that can cause a "high order of destruction." The intentional use of these weapons must cause mass casualties, defined as more than 1,000 injured or dead, during a single incident.

A disaster is a sudden, calamitous event that seriously disrupts the functioning of a community or society and causes human, material, and economic or environmental losses that exceed the community's or society's ability to cope using its own resources. This scenario can develop increasing complexity due to the potentially disorganized egress of the population in combination with the response from multiple agencies—most urgently, fire, police, and emergency medical services (EMS). Access is a challenge, and establishment of incident command is a priority. Designating a staging area; delineating hot, warm, and cold zones; and establishing a safe corridor to operate are all priorities for incident command at a potential radiologic emergency.

Initial Assessment of the Incident

Because this scenario is for a nonaccidental explosion, police may be the lead agency in some municipalities. Alternatively, reports that casualties are rising may necessitate the establishment of unified command, with an incident command structure that includes more than one agency. Given the alarming dosimeters, the fire service and hazardous materials teams will play an instrumental role, and establishment of patient decontamination may become a priority. EMS will be required for patient treatment and transport. EMS personnel must be familiar with the operational priorities at a CBRN event in order to operate safely, with awareness of the appropriate personal protective equipment (PPE) and precautions.

Types of Radiologic Incidents

There are four types of weapons that can cause a radiologic incident:

1. **Radiologic dispersal device (RDD).** A conventional explosive device with radiologic contaminants present or any device that can disperse radioactive material. Contamination will vary by device and source. The number of victims resulting from use of this type of device can vary from small to large.
2. **Radiologic exposure device (RED).** A simple radiologic device designed to expose people to radiation only, with no contamination present. Use of this type of device results in an incident with a small number of victims.
3. **Radiologic incendiary device (RID).** This type of device increases panic by pairing fire with radioactive contamination.
4. **Improvised nuclear device (IND).** INDs are illicit nuclear weapons bought, stolen, or otherwise originating from a nuclear state. They can also be a weapon fabricated by a terrorist group from illegally obtained fissile nuclear weapons material that produces a nuclear explosion. Incidents from this type of device result in a large number of victims.

CBRN Abbreviation for the constellation of chemical, biologic, radiologic, and nuclear hazards.

weapon of mass destruction (WMD) A nuclear, biologic, or chemical weapon that can cause a high order of destruction.

disaster A sudden, calamitous event that seriously disrupts the functioning of a community or society and causes human, material, and economic or environmental losses that exceed the community's or society's ability to cope using its own resources.

radiologic dispersal device (RDD) A conventional explosive device with radiologic contaminants present, or any device that can disperse radioactive material.

radiologic exposure device (RED) A simple radiologic device designed to expose people to radiation.

radiologic incendiary device (RID) A radiologic device pairing fire with radioactive contamination.

improvised nuclear device (IND) An illicit nuclear weapon bought, stolen, or otherwise originating from a nuclear state, or a weapon fabricated by a terrorist group from illegally obtained fissile nuclear weapons material that produces a nuclear explosion.

The Worried Well

Following a CBRN event, many people who were exposed to minimal CBRN agent, or none at all, will seek medical care and slow down medical treatment of genuinely affected patients. These worried well patients may compose up to 20 times the number of injured or affected patients and may become one of the most difficult aspects in dealing with WMD events. In the 1995 Tokyo sarin gas event, 85% of those seeking treatment were the worried well.

CHECK YOUR KNOWLEDGE

A priority for the initial incident commander at a radiologic event is to:

A. identify a holding area for the worried well.
B. delineate hot, warm, and cold zones.
C. determine the type of device involved.
D. establish a media liaison position.

Radiation Physics

Radiation is the process by which energy is emitted as particles or waves. Whole-body exposure to ionizing radiation is measured in terms of the **gray (Gy)**. The radiation absorbed dose, or rad, was a familiar dose unit that was replaced by the gray; 1 Gy equals 100 rad. The roentgen equivalent man (rem) describes the dose in rad multiplied by a quality factor, which takes into account the intrinsic special deposition pattern of different types of radiation. The rem has been replaced with the **sievert (Sv)**; 1 Sv equals 100 rem.

Types of Ionizing Radiation

Alpha particles are relatively large and cannot penetrate even a few layers of skin. Intact skin or a uniform offers adequate protection from external contamination-emitting alpha particles. Ionizing radiation from alpha particles is a concern only if it is internalized in the body by inhaling or ingesting alpha-particle emitters. When internalized, alpha-particle radiation can cause significant local cellular injury to adjacent cells.

Beta particles are small charged particles that can penetrate more deeply than alpha particles can. They can affect deeper levels of skin and can injure the base of the skin, causing a beta burn. Beta-particle radiation is found most frequently in nuclear fallout. Beta particles also result in local radiation injury.

Gamma radiation, much like X-rays, can easily penetrate tissue. Gamma rays are emitted with a nuclear detonation and fallout. They could also be emitted from some radionuclides that might be present in an RDD. Gamma radiation can result in a whole-body exposure, which can result in acute and chronic radiation sickness.

Neutron radiation can penetrate tissue easily, with 20 times the destructive energy of gamma rays, disrupting the atomic structure of cells. Neutrons are released during a nuclear explosion but are not a fallout risk. Neutrons also contribute to whole-body radiation exposure and can result in acute radiation sickness. **FIGURE 2-1** shows the various types of ionizing radiation.

worried well People who do not need medical treatment but who seek it for the sake of being reassured.

gray (Gy) A unit used to measure whole-body exposure to ionizing radiation. 1 Gy = 100 rad.

sievert (Sv) A unit of dose equivalent (the biologic effect of ionizing radiation), equal to an effective dose of a joule of energy per kilogram of recipient mass. 1 Sv = 100 rem.

alpha particle A particle with two neutrons and two protons that is ejected from the nucleus of a radioactive atom. The particle is identical to the nucleus of a helium atom.

beta particle A high-energy, high-speed electron emitted from the nucleus of a radioactive atom and most frequently found in nuclear fallout. Because this electron is from the nucleus of the atom, it is called a beta particle to distinguish it from the electrons that orbit the atom.

gamma radiation Penetrating electromagnetic radiation of a kind arising from the radioactive decay of atomic nuclei.

neutron radiation A kind of ionizing radiation that consists of free neutrons. Free neutrons are released from atoms as a result of nuclear fission or nuclear fusion and then react with nuclei of other atoms to form new isotopes, which, in turn, may produce radiation.

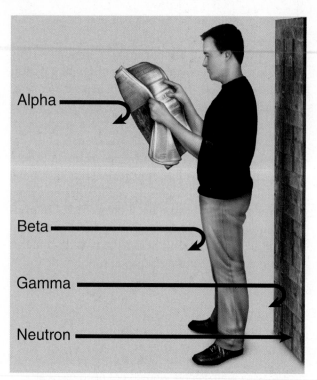

Figure 2-1 Types of ionizing radiation.
© Jones & Bartlett Learning.

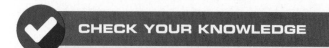
CHECK YOUR KNOWLEDGE

The most dangerous type of ionizing radiation is:

A. neutron radiation.
B. gamma radiation.
C. beta-particle radiation.
D. alpha-particle radiation.

radiation sickness Damage to the body caused by a large dose of radiation often received over a short period (acute). The amount of radiation absorbed by the body—the absorbed dose—determines how sick the patient will be.

acute radiation syndrome A serious illness that can result from exposure to very high levels of radiation, usually over a short period. The amount of radiation that a person's body absorbs is called the radiation dose.

Radiation Pathophysiology

Radiation causes ionizations in the molecules of living cells. These ionizations result in the removal of electrons from the atoms, forming ions (i.e., charged atoms). The ions formed can go on to react with other atoms in the cell, causing damage. For example, if a gamma ray passes through a cell, the water molecules near the DNA might be ionized, and the ions might react with the DNA, causing it to break. At low doses, such as what we receive every day from background radiation, the cells repair the damage rapidly. At higher doses, the cells might not be able to repair the damage, and the cells may either be changed permanently or die. Most cells that die are of little consequence; the body can simply replace them. Cells changed permanently may produce abnormal cells when they divide. In the right circumstance, these cells may become cancerous. Thus, increased radiation exposure can increase risk of cancer.

Radiation effects occur at the cellular level. Cells that are actively dividing are more sensitive to radiation. Examples include blood-forming cells, sperm cells, hair follicles, gastrointestinal cells, and embryonic cells. The effects of radiation on these cells are commonly seen in patients undergoing chemotherapy. Injury may also occur from physical properties of the radioactive source. Some radioactive materials are corrosive, flammable, or toxic and can pose a contact hazard.

Acute Radiation Dose

At even higher doses, cells cannot be replaced fast enough, and tissues fail to function. An example of this process is radiation sickness. Radiation sickness results after high doses to the whole body, in which the intestinal lining is damaged to the point that it cannot perform its functions of processing water and nutrients and protecting the body against infection. This impaired intestinal functioning leads to nausea, diarrhea, and general weakness. With higher whole-body doses, the body's immune system is damaged and cannot fight off infection and disease.

Immediate biologic effects from an acute dose can include radiation burns or, with greater doses, radiation syndrome. Symptoms of acute radiation syndrome include nausea, vomiting, diarrhea, fatigue, hair loss, and decreased organ function. Although exposure to radiation can cause burns to the skin, radiation does not appear instantaneously, and a large absorbed dose is required for radiation burns to occur at all. Burns that develop on scene rather than hours or days later may be chemical or thermal in nature (**TABLE 2-1**).

Chronic Radiation Dose

While the body is better able to handle smaller doses of radiation over a long period, allowing for time to replace or repair

TABLE 2-1 Acute Radiation Syndrome

Feature	Effects of Whole-Body Irradiation or Internal Absorption, by Dose Range in rad (1 rad = 1 centigray; 100 rad = 1 gray)					
	0–100 (0–1 Gy)	100–200 (1–2 Gy)	200–600 (2–6 Gy)	600–800 (6–8 Gy)	800–3,000 (8–30 Gy)	>3,000 (>30 Gy)
Prodromal Phase of Syndrome						
Nausea, vomiting	None	5–50%	50–100%	75–100%	90–100%	100%
Time of onset	—	3–6 hr	2–4 hr	1–2 hr	< 1 hr	N/A
Duration	—	< 24 hr	< 24 hr	< 48 hr	48 hr	N/A
Lymphocyte count	Unaffected	Minimally decreased	< 1,000 at 24 hr	< 500 at 24 hr	Decreases within hours	Decreases within hours
CNS function	No impairment	No impairment	Routine task performance Cognitive impairment for 6–20 hr	Simple, routine task performance Cognitive impairment for > 24 hr	Rapid incapacitation; May have a lucid interval of several hours	
Latent Phase of Syndrome						
No symptoms	> 2 wk	7–15 d	0–7 d	0–2 d	None	None

(continues)

TABLE 2-1 Acute Radiation Syndrome *(continued)*

Feature	0–100 (0–1 Gy)	100–200 (1–2 Gy)	200–600 (2–6 Gy)	600–800 (6–8 Gy)	800–3,000 (8–30 Gy)	> 3,000 (> 30 Gy)
Effects of Whole-Body Irradiation or Internal Absorption, by Dose Range in rad (1 rad = 1 centigray; 100 rad = 1 gray)						
Manifest Illness						
Signs/ symptoms	None	Moderate leukopenia	Severe leukopenia, purpura, hemorrhage, pneumonia, hair loss after 300 rad		Diarrhea, fever, electrolyte disturbance	Convulsions, ataxia, tremor, lethargy
Time of onset	—	> 2 wk	2 d to 4 wk	2 d to 4 wk	1–3 d	1–3 d
Critical period	—	None	4–6 wk; greatest potential for effective medical intervention		2–14 d	1–46 hr
Organ system	None	—	Hematopoietic; respiratory (mucosal) systems		GI tract Mucosal systems	CNS
Hospitalization duration	0%	< 5% 45–60 d	90% 60–90 d	100% 100+ d	100% Weeks to months	100% Days to weeks
Mortality	None	Minimal	Low with aggressive therapy	High	Very high; significant neurologic symptoms indicate lethal dose	

CNS, central nervous system; d, day(s); hr, hour(s); N/A, not available; wk, week(s).

Modified from Armed Forces Radiobiology Research Institute: Medical management of radiological casualties, Bethesda, MD, 2003.

damaged cells, a **chronic radiation dose** may suppress the immune system and predispose it to bacterial, viral, or fungal opportunistic infections. Chronic exposure does not produce the immediate physical effects seen with an acute dose. Victims may develop cancer, leukemia, bone destruction, and mutations. These changes can potentially be passed to offspring if damage has occurred in germ cells.

Radiation, unlike chemical exposure, is a carcinogen without a definitive threshold. Many factors are involved in determining a person's risk of developing cancer, including cumulative dose of radiation, the duration of exposure, genetic factors, a person's lifestyle and health, and a host of other factors.

CHECK YOUR KNOWLEDGE

Diarrhea, hair loss, and decreased organ function are symptoms of:

A. chronic radiation exposure.
B. fifth-degree radiation burn.
C. radiation syndrome.
D. worried well psychosis.

EMS Response to a Radiologic Event

EMS providers must ensure they have and properly use all PPE when operating at a radiologic event. Respiratory protection is essential to avoid injury from exposure to alpha or beta radiation. Self-contained breathing apparatus (SCBA) are required when operating in the hot zone.

When all hazards are identified and the work area has sufficient oxygen, the incident commander may decide that members can operate with air-purifying respirators (APRs), powered air-purifying respirators (PAPRs), or N95 filtering face-piece respiratory masks. The APR may be particularly useful to rescuers whose SCBA tank is near empty and who are out of the immediate hazard area or out of an area requiring full bunker gear and respiratory protection; the APR is suitable protection for most radiologic emergencies. Emergencies involving other hazards, such as an **immediately dangerous to life and health (IDLH)** environment (i.e., chemicals, vapors, low oxygen), require SCBA and additional PPE. Each member must don a dosimeter when operating at a radiologic emergency.

Dose Versus Rate of Exposure

It is vital to understand the difference between **dose** and **dose rate**. Any readings relayed to the incident division,

branch, or group commander must include the appropriate units (e.g., mR or rem versus mR/h or rem/h). The dose a member will receive operating for the duration of one SCBA bottle, which will last less than 30 minutes, will be less than the rate number on the meter's readout. For example, a person operating in an environment with a meter reading of 50 mR/h will receive a dose of 50 mR if operating for 1 hour in that environment, or 25 mR if operating for half an hour.

Dose, as it relates to radiation exposure, is the amount of radiation energy deposited or absorbed in the body. It is measured in microrem (μR), millirem (mR), or rem (1,000,000 μR = 1,000 mR = 1 rem) using a dosimeter. Common dosimeters include the Science Applications International Corporation (SAIC) pager dosimeter and the Canberra UltraRadiac.

Rate of exposure (dose-rate) identifies how fast the radiation energy is deposited. The dose-rate is measured in microrem/h (μR/h), millirem/h (mR/h), or rem/h. Common devices used to read dose-rate include the Radalert 50 (mR/h range), Ludlum Models 23 or 25 (rem/h range), or Canberra UltraRadiac (mR/h and rem/h).

CHECK YOUR KNOWLEDGE

The amount of radiation energy deposited or absorbed in the body is identified as the:

A. dose.
B. mR/h.
C. dose rate.
D. IDLH exposure.

chronic radiation dose A dose of ionizing radiation received either continuously or intermittently over a prolonged period.

immediately dangerous to life and health (IDLH) Defined by the U.S. National Institute for Occupational Safety and Health as exposure to airborne contaminants that is "likely to cause death or immediate or delayed permanent adverse health effects or prevent escape from such an environment."

dose The amount of radiation energy deposited or absorbed in the body.

dose rate A measurement of how fast the radiation energy is deposited; also known as rate of exposure.

Radiation Measuring Devices

Devices commonly used to measure radiation include the following (**FIGURE 2-2**):

- The Radalert 50 carried on department apparatus is calibrated to alarm at 1 mR/h.
- The Radalert 50 can measure radiation levels up to 50 mR/h. This rate is well below the rate at which signs and symptoms of acute radiation exposure are observable.
- The Ludlum models, carried by many hazardous materials units, can read up to 100 rem/h.
- The SAIC dosimeters and Canberra UltraRadiacs can read up to 999 rem/h.

CHECK YOUR KNOWLEDGE

The Radalert 50, a radiation measuring device commonly used by EMS responders, is calibrated to alarm at:

A. 100 rem/h.
B. 50 mR/h.
C. 20 mR/h.
D. 1 mR/h.

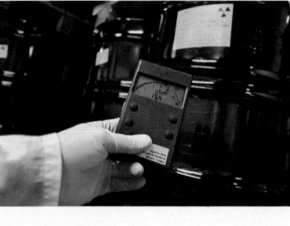

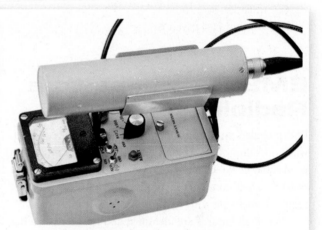

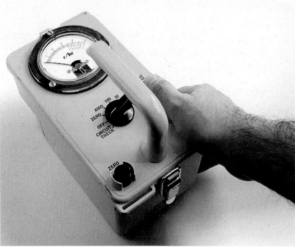

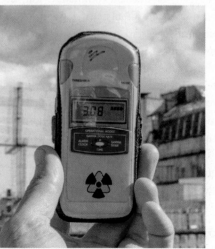

Figure 2-2 Types of radiation monitoring devices.

Initial Management of a Radiologic Incident

Approaching an incident involving a radioactive material is not significantly different from approaching an incident involving other hazardous materials. Attempt to approach the incident scene from upwind and uphill, and try to identify the hazard from as far away as possible, using binoculars if available. Identify the source of the radiation and the conditions surrounding the incident, such as the integrity of any containers or packages or other factors. Make appropriate notifications and, if needed, initiate the incident command system.

Use Guide 163: Radioactive Materials (Low to High Level Radiation) of the *Emergency Response Guide* (*EGR*) to determine your isolation distances, starting with an initial area of 75 feet (23 m) in all directions. Note that the *EGR* states, "Medical problems take priority over radiological concerns." Radiologic events require focus on three items for provider safety:

1. Minimize your time in the hot zone.
2. Maintain a safe distance from radioactive materials.
3. Use shielding whenever possible.

Always procure your radiation detection equipment and zero-out the meter.

Intentional Impact of Radiation Release by Device

Radiologic Dispersal Device

Characteristics of RDDs include the following:

- Disperse radioactive material as a solid (powder), liquid (mist), or a gas over a large area
- Can involve explosives and are also known as "dirty bombs"
- Result in above-background radiologic meter readings at multiple locations
- Cause contamination (therefore, internal and external exposures should be expected)

Radiologic Exposure Device

Characteristics of REDs include the following:

- Involve a point source intended to expose a specific person or population to doses of radiation
- Cause a smaller, more limited hot zone than results from RDDs

- May be secretly hidden, thereby delaying recognition or identification of the emergency
- Do not cause contamination if radioactive material is contained (therefore, external exposure only should be expected)

Radiologic Incendiary Device

Characteristics of RIDs include the following:

- Involve radiologic material in an intentionally set fire (sometimes called a "dirty fire")
- Are used in a type of attack to deliberately delay first responders
- Pose the greatest danger from the expanding fire
- Cause contamination with potential internal and external exposures

Improvised Nuclear Device

Characteristics of INDs include the following:

- Result in high levels of radiation and contamination
- Result in extensive casualties with multiple types of injuries
- Result in higher doses of internal and external radiation
- Present such catastrophic potential that operations must be modified

Incident Command for a Radiologic Event

The initial scene size-up includes determining the number of injured and exposed or contaminated individuals. Based on the type of device and event, determine the type of injuries requiring intervention. As soon as possible, document the radiation level in the area to identify the hot, warm, and cold zones.

To form the incident action plan (IAP), many factors must be known. The presence of other hazards at the event, such a fire, chemical, explosive, or asphyxiant, will determine the level of PPE needed by the emergency responders. The IAP also requires determination of whether the atmosphere in the work area is IDLH and whether a secondary device or other threats to responders exist. The IAP will outline the risk versus benefit parameters (**TABLE 2-2**).

Managing Life Hazards

There are four activities in managing life hazards at a radiologic event:

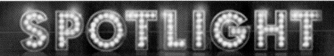

Level A and Level B PPE

- Level A:
  - Totally encapsulated chemical and vapor-protective suit
  - Chemical-resistant inner suit
  - Positive-pressure full face-piece SCBA or supplied air respirator
  - Inner and outer chemical-resistant gloves and chemical-resistant safety boots
  - Maximum available skin, respiratory, and eye protection
- Level B:
  - Hooded chemical-resistant clothing
  - Chemical-resistant inner suit
  - Positive-pressure full face-piece SCBA or supplied air respirator
  - Inner and outer chemical-resistant gloves and chemical-resistant safety boots

TABLE 2-2 Risk Versus Benefit Parameters	
Decision Dose (whole body)	**Emergency Activity Performed**
50 rem	Lifesaving for a catastrophic event
25 rem	Lifesaving or protection of large populations
10 rem	Protections of major property
5 rem	General operations at a radiological emergency

© Jones & Bartlett Learning.

1. **Isolate.** Establish an area and restrict access to the hot zone. Create zones to prevent spread of contamination and/or cross-contamination. EMS providers must not proceed into the hot zone except for lifesaving purposes, such as rescue and recon or fire suppression.
2. **Contain.** Protect surrounding structures from contamination by shutting down the heating, ventilation, and air conditioning outside air intakes until the presence and extent of radioactive material are evaluated.
3. **Evacuate.** Move civilians from the surrounding area if the projected dose inside the building will reach 5 rem for the general population or 10 rem for institutional residents, such as nursing home residents, prison inmates, and nonambulatory hospital patients. If time permits, evacuate civilians before a radioactive plume arrives.

4. **Shelter-in-place.** Shelter-in-place is a viable option if rapid evacuation is impeded or not feasible. Building materials provide substantial radiation protection; relying on this level of protection may be safer than evacuating through a contaminated area.

 CHECK YOUR KNOWLEDGE

When would an EMS provider proceed into the hot zone?

A. To determine the type of device that is emitting radioactivity.
B. To retrieve a transport manifest or related identification documents.
C. To complete a lifesaving activity.
D. A provider will never proceed into the hot zone.

Establishing the Hot, Warm, and Cold Zones

Hot Zone: Greater Than 2 mR/h

The hotline is established at 2 mR/h. Victims being removed from the hot zone to the warm zone may have levels of radiation greater than 2 mR/h before they are decontaminated. The hotline is the edge of the hot zone and the point beyond which no contamination is present (i.e., area is cold). This rate is also established to restrict unnecessary access to highly contaminated areas during the response but still allows access for emergency workers performing life safety operations and protection of major property. Hot zone activities are restricted to rescue and fire suppression activities, and ambulatory victims are directed to the warm zone for decontamination.

Warm Zone: 2 mR/h

The warm zone is established if contamination is present and decontamination procedures need to be implemented. The warm zone provides a safe refuge area (SRA) in which assessment for trauma and decontamination by EMS occur. Proper decontamination of victims should be verified before victims are directed to the cold zone for retriage, treatment, and transport.

Cold Zone: Less Than 2 mR/h

Support operations and command are based in the cold zone.

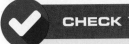

CHECK YOUR KNOWLEDGE

A safe refuge area has a radiation level of:
A. 2 mR/h.
B. between 4 mR/h and 2.01 mR/h.
C. over 4 mR/h.
D. less than 2 mR/h.

Decontamination

After determining the number of victims, a decontamination process for civilians and responders is established in the warm zone, and the proper level of PPE for those performing the decontamination process is selected

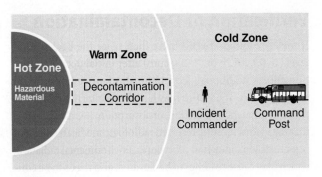

Figure 2-3 The decontamination corridor.
© Jones & Bartlett Learning.

(**FIGURE 2-3**). Factors in selecting the decontamination corridor include proximity to the incident, wind direction, terrain, and water runoff.

Factors influencing the priority for decontamination include the following:

1. Patients with life-threatening injuries (i.e., injuries that affect airway, breathing, and circulation [ABCs])
2. Patients that are most severely contaminated but are not symptomatic
3. Discretion should be used to prioritize the remaining contaminated patients:
   - Pregnant women
   - Children
   - Senior citizens
   - Non-life-threatening injuries

Dry decontamination is the preferred method for radiologic events, followed by limited amounts of washing (face, hair, hands, feet). Dry decontamination relies on the physical removal of radioactive contamination by removing clothing and/or brushing or removing contaminants from the clothing with tape. A large percentage of contamination can be eliminated with the removal of victim's outer clothing (depending on the season and amount of clothing worn). There are five types of dry decontamination, each of which can be used in conjunction with the other types to remove up to 100% of all suspected contaminants:

1. Scraping
2. Adsorbent materials
3. Absorbent materials
4. Vacuuming
5. Pressurized air

Wet decontamination may be needed for large-scale radiologic emergencies, because it is a quick way to deal with extensive external contamination. Weather and air or water temperature are limiting factors.

Verification of Decontamination

If meter readings are still more than twice the background level (> 0.1 mR/h or > 200 cpm) after initial decontamination efforts, additional decontamination procedures should be considered. The victim may have been internally exposed through inhalation, ingestion, or absorption. It is also possible that the victim recently received radiologic medical treatment prior to decontamination procedures. Environmental radiation, which may cause readings to be elevated, also needs to be considered. If environmental radiation levels are elevated, direct the meter's probe closer to the victim to get a more accurate reading of radiation levels being emitted from the person.

 CHECK YOUR KNOWLEDGE

A patient who has undergone initial decontamination requires additional decontamination procedures if he or she is still showing meter readings that are more than _____ times the level of background radiation.

A. 10.2
B. 7.5
C. 2.0
D. 1.2

SUMMARY

- A disaster is a sudden, calamitous event that seriously disrupts the functioning of a community or society and causes human, material, and economic or environmental losses that exceed the community's or society's ability to cope using its own resources.
- There are four types of weapons that can cause a radiologic incident: radiologic dispersion device (RDD), radiologic exposure device (RED), radiologic incendiary device (RID), and improvised nuclear device (IND).
- Radiation is the process by which energy is emitted as particles or waves. Types of ionizing radiation include alpha-particle, beta-particle, gamma, and neutron radiation.
- Radiation causes ionizations in the molecules of living cells. These ionizations result in the removal of electrons from the atoms, forming ions (i.e., charged atoms), which can go on to react with other atoms in the cell, causing damage.
- EMS providers must ensure they have and properly use all PPE when operating at a radiologic event.
- Dose is the amount of radiation energy deposited or absorbed in the body, and the dose-rate or rate of exposure identifies how fast the radiation energy is deposited.
- Devices commonly used to measure radiation include the Radalert 50, Ludlum models, SAIC dosimeters, and the Canberra UltraRadiac.
- Approaching an incident involving a radioactive material is not significantly different from approaching an incident involving other hazardous materials. Attempt to approach the incident scene from upwind and uphill, and try to identify the hazard from as far away as possible, using binoculars if available. Identify the source of the radiation and the conditions surrounding the incident, such as the integrity of any containers or packages or other factors.
- Hot zone activities are restricted to rescue and fire suppression activities. The warm zone is established if contamination is present. It provides a safe refuge area (SRA) in which assessment for trauma and decontamination by EMS occur. Support operations and command are based in the cold zone. Proper decontamination of victims should be verified before victims are directed to the cold zone for retriage, treatment, and transport.
- After determining the number of victims, a decontamination process for civilians and responders is established in the warm zone, and the proper level of PPE for those performing the decontamination process is selected. Factors in selecting the decontamination corridor include proximity to the incident, wind direction, terrain, and water runoff.

REFERENCES AND ADDITIONAL RESOURCES

Department of Energy Office of Transportation and Emergency Management. (2007, January). *Model procedures for first responder initial response to radiolological transportation accidents* (Rev. 4). Washington, DC: Transportation Emergency Preparedness Program (TEPP). Retrieved from https://energy.gov/sites/prod/files/em/TEPP/2-b-1FirstResponderInitialResponse.pdf

Federal Emergency Management Agency. (2013). *National response framework* (2nd ed.). Washington, DC: U.S. Department of Homeland Security.

Incident and Emergency Centre. (2006, October). *Manual for first responders to a radiological emergency.* Vienna, Austria: International Atomic Energy Agency. Retrieved from http://www-pub.iaea.org/mtcd/publications/pdf/epr_firstresponder_web.pdf

Los Angeles County Emergency Medical Services Agency. (2013, October 30). *Ambulance guidelines for response to radiation events* (Rev. 7). Los Angeles, CA: Los Angeles County Department of Health Services. Retrieved from http://file.lacounty.gov/SDSInter/dhs/216885_AmbulanceGuidelinesforResponsetoRadiationEventsRev7-20131030.pdf

Mauroni, A. (2010, September). Homeland insecurity: Thinking about CBRN terrorism. *Homeland Security Affairs, 6*, Article 3. Retrieved from https://www.hsaj.org/articles/78

Pipeline and Hazardous Materials Safety Administration. (2016). *2016 emergency response guidebook.* Washington, DC: U.S. Department of Transportation. Retrieved from http://www.phmsa.dot.gov/staticfiles/PHMSA/DownloadableFiles/Files/Hazmat/ERG2016.pdf

Stone, F. P. (2007, June). *The "worried well" response to CBRN events: Analysis and solutions: Counter proliferation paper number 40.* Maxwell Air Force Base, AL: USAF Counterproliferation Center. Retrieved from https://fas.org/irp/threat/cbw/worried.pdf

U.S. Department of Health and Human Services. (n.d.). First responders in the field. Radiation Emergency Medical Management. Retrieved from https://www.remm.nlm.gov/remm_FirstResponder.htm

CRITICAL THINKING SKILL STATION

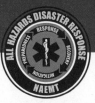

Practitioner Preparedness Self-Assessment

Exercise Introduction: The purpose of this exercise is for you to assess and improve your ability to continue to perform your duties as an EMS practitioner during a disaster affecting your community.

How many days of food and water do you have readily available in your household?

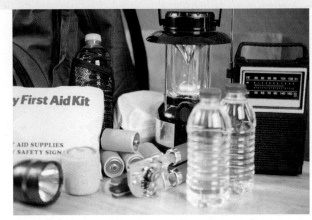

© fstop123/iStock/Getty.

- Store at least 1 gallon of water per day for each person and each pet. You should consider storing more water than this for hot climates, for pregnant women, and for persons who are sick.
- Store at least a 3-day supply of water for each person and each pet. Try to store a 2-week supply, if possible.
- Try to store at least a 3-day supply of food per family, including pets. Remember, it is better to have extra food that you can share than to run out of food during an emergency.
- Choose foods that last a long time, do not need to be refrigerated, and are easy to make.
- Make sure you have a manual can opener and disposable utensils.

If you have children, who would care for them if you needed to serve extended tours of duty?

If you have pets, who would care for them if you needed to serve extended tours of duty?

What emergency supplies should you keep in your household?

- Prescription medications and glasses
- Infant formula and diapers
- Pet food and extra water for your pet
- Important family documents such as copies of insurance policies, identification, and bank account records in a waterproof, portable container
- Cash or traveler's checks and change
- Sleeping bag or warm blanket for each person. Consider additional bedding if you live in a cold-weather climate.
- Complete change of clothing including a long-sleeved shirt, long pants, and sturdy shoes. Consider additional clothing if you live in a cold-weather climate.
- Household chlorine bleach and medicine dropper. Bleach can be used as a disinfectant when diluted nine parts water to one part bleach. In an emergency, you can use regular household bleach to treat water by using 16 drops per gallon of water. Do not use scented or color-safe bleach, or bleaches with added cleaners.
- Fire extinguisher
- Matches in a waterproof container
- Feminine supplies and personal hygiene items
- Mess kits, paper cups, plates and plastic utensils, and paper towels
- Manual can opener
- Paper and pencil
- Books, games, puzzles, or other activities for children

3 Natural Disasters and Infrastructure Failures

OBJECTIVES

After studying this chapter, you will be able to:

- Identify reasons to shelter-in-place.

- Identify alternative transport considerations during a disaster.

- Discuss the importance of patient tracking during an evacuation, and explain how it is accomplished.

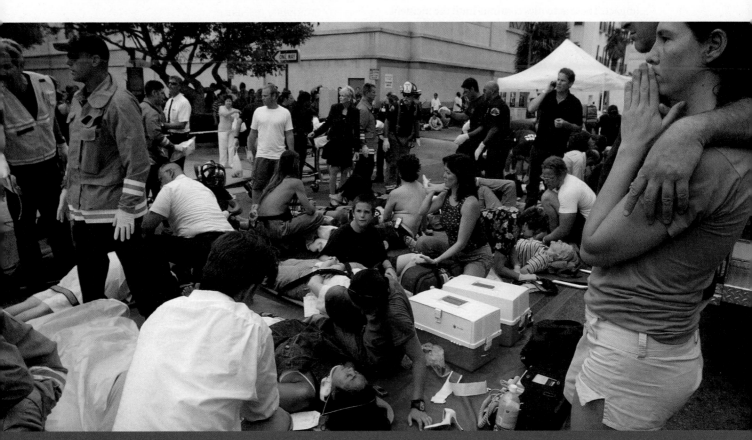

The Disaster Cycle

Eric Noji and other disaster response experts have defined a framework to analyze and prepare for a disaster. A disaster can be broken down into five phases:

1. **Quiescence phase or interdisaster phase**. This phase is the time in between disasters or mass-casualty incidents during which risk assessment and mitigation activities should be performed. This is the period to practice response and disaster implementation training and deployment exercises.

2. **Prodrome phase or warning phase**. This phase focuses on a specific event that has been identified as inevitable, such as an incoming hurricane or an imminent failure of an element of the infrastructure. During this predisaster period, steps may be taken to mitigate the effects of the ensuing events. These steps include mobilizing resources, fortifying physical structures, and initiating evacuation plans.

3. **Impact phase**. This phase is the occurrence of the actual event. Little can be done during the impact phase to alter the effects or outcome of what is occurring.

4. **Response phase**. This phase activates the emergency services, rescue, and relief operations needed to save lives and preserve communities after the impact. These activities continue until the incident commander declares the event "under control."

5. **Recovery and reconstruction phase**. During this phase, community resources are used to endure, emerge from, and rebuild after the effects of the disaster through the coordinated efforts of medical, public health, and community infrastructure. Following massive disasters, such as Hurricane Sandy in 2012, the recovery and reconstruction stage may take years.

Emergency management planning involves four phases:

1. Mitigation
2. Planning
3. Response
4. Recovery

Some authorities may include a fifth phase, prevention. With each lesson learned from a major event, the emergency management process is updated. **FIGURE 3-1** shows the relationships among the event, emergency management planning, and the disaster cycle.

CHECK YOUR KNOWLEDGE

The _____ phase of the disaster cycle is when EMS providers can make the biggest contribution to community resilience.

A. quiescence
B. prodrome
C. response
D. recovery and reconstruction

---

quiescence phase The time in between disasters or mass-casualty incidents during which risk assessment and mitigation activities should be performed.

prodrome phase Preparation for a specific event that has been identified as inevitable, such as an incoming hurricane or an imminent failure of an element of the infrastructure.

impact phase The occurrence of an actual event, such as a hurricane or mass-casualty incident.

response phase The emergency services rescue and relief operations to save lives and preserve communities after the impact of an event.

recovery and reconstruction phase Use of community resources to endure, emerge from, and rebuild after the effects of a disaster.

evacuation The rapid movement of people away from the immediate threat or impact of a disaster to a safer place of shelter.

Situations That Require Evacuation

The purpose of evacuations is to save and protect the lives of people exposed to actual or imminent danger through their timely and rapid movement to safer locations and places of shelter. With the threat and impact of natural disasters such as severe storms, floods, earthquakes, and wild fires, hundreds to millions of people may need to move within a very short period. **Evacuation** is the rapid movement of people away from the immediate threat or impact of a disaster to a safer place of shelter. It is commonly characterized by a short time frame, from hours to weeks, within which emergency procedures need to be enacted to save lives and minimize exposure to harm.

People displaced from their homes or places of habitual residence by disasters, including evacuees, often face risks due to their displacement. International research shows that

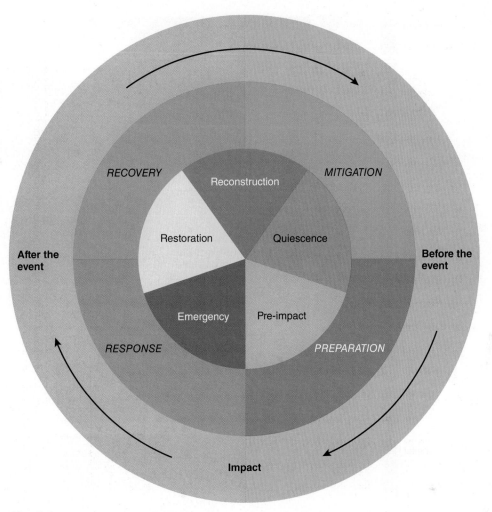

Figure 3-1 The disaster cycle.

Data from Alexander, David. 2002. *Principles of Emergency Planning and Management*. Oxford: Oxford University Press.

long-term psychological and social harm is often caused to individuals after evacuation, particularly in cases where evacuees are unable to return to their original homes. Compared to others affected by an emergency but who are not dislocated from their homes and communities, evacuees can suffer up to twice the rate of illness.

Phases of Evacuation

The Post-Katrina Emergency Management Reform Act of 2006 authorizes the use of Urban Area Security Initiative or Homeland Security Grant program funds for states to develop catastrophic mass evacuation plans. A state-level plan notes that the local jurisdiction impacted by the natural disaster or infrastructure failure will make the decision to begin an evacuation as prescribed in local laws, policies, and authority. The decision to evacuate will depend on the nature, scope, and severity of the emergency; the number of people affected; and the actions necessary to protect the public.

In deciding whether to evacuate or shelter-in-place, the timing and nature of the incident must be carefully considered. Because evacuation is an effective means of moving people out of a dangerous area, preparation for evacuation should be an immediate consideration. However, owing to its complexity and the stress it puts on the population, evacuation may not be the best option when other viable options are available. The phases of an evacuation include the evacuation warning and an immediate evacuation order (**FIGURE 3-2**).

- **Evacuation warning.** *Evacuation warning* is the official term for the alert issued to people in an affected area of a potential threat to life and property.

evacuation warning The alert issued to people in an affected area of a potential threat to life and property.

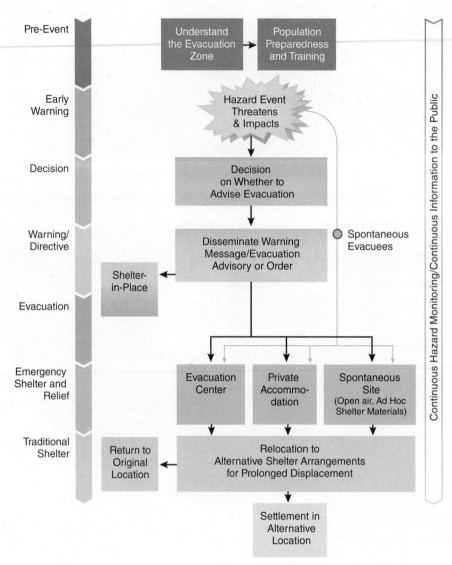

Figure 3-2 Evacuation phases.

Data from Internal Displacement Monitoring Centre (2013) *Global Estimates 2012: People Displaced by Disasters.*

People who need additional time should consider evacuating when the warning is issued rather than waiting for an immediate evacuation order. An evacuation warning considers the probability that an area will be affected and prepares people for a potential immediate evacuation order. This warning is often associated with the term *voluntary evacuation* by the media.

immediate evacuation order An order requiring the immediate movement of people out of an affected area due to an imminent threat to life.

- **Immediate evacuation order.** An immediate evacuation order requires the immediate movement of people out of an affected area due to an imminent threat to life. Choosing to stay could result in loss of life and could impede the work of emergency personnel. In a rapidly developing emergency, an immediate evacuation order may be the only warning that people in the affected area receive. This order is often associated with the term *mandatory evacuation* by the media. The evacuation announcement should involve activation of the Emergency Alert System, use of traditional media, use of social media, and door-to-door messaging.

Shelter-in-Place Versus Evacuation

To **shelter-in-place** may become the preferred option to avoid exposure to outside environmental hazards, such as radiologic or airborne contaminants. The decision to shelter-in-place requires an organized method of securing building entrances, including windows and ventilation systems, to prevent outside environmental hazards from entering the building. Building and safety personnel, homeowners, and residents should have contingencies to move to and/or create safe rooms and designated safe areas if sheltering-in-place is recommended.

Vulnerable Patients

The National Response Framework (NRF) provides a function-based approach to address the needs of vulnerable patients. The NRF defines members of a **special needs population** as individuals with needs before, during, and after an incident in the following functional areas:

- **Maintaining independence.** Individuals requiring support to be independent in daily activities may lose this support during the course of an emergency or a disaster. This support may include supplies (e.g., diapers, formula, catheters, ostomy supplies), durable medical equipment (e.g., wheelchairs, walkers, and scooters), and/or attendants or caregivers. Supplying needed support to these individuals will enable them to maintain their predisaster level of independence.
- **Communication.** Individuals who have limitations that interfere with the receipt of and response to information will need that information provided in methods they can understand and use. They may not be able to hear verbal announcements, see directional signs, or understand how to get assistance because of hearing, vision, speech, cognitive, and/or intellectual limitations, and/or limited English proficiency.
- **Transportation.** Individuals who cannot drive or who do not have a vehicle may require transportation support for successful evacuation. This support may include accessible vehicles (e.g., lift-equipped vehicles, vehicles suitable for transporting individuals who use oxygen) or information about how and where to access mass transportation during an evacuation.
- **Supervision.** Before, during, and after an emergency, individuals may lose the support of caregivers, family, or friends or may be unable to cope in a new environment (particularly if they have dementia or psychiatric conditions such as schizophrenia or intense anxiety). If separated from their caregivers, young children may be unable to identify themselves and, when in danger, may lack the cognitive ability to assess the situation and react appropriately.
- **Medical care.** Individuals who are not self-sufficient or who do not have adequate support from caregivers, family, or friends may need assistance with

shelter-in-place Selecting a small, interior room, with no or few windows, and taking refuge there.

special needs population Groups whose needs are not fully addressed by traditional service providers or who feel they cannot comfortably or safely access and use the standard resources offered in disaster preparedness, relief, and recovery.

managing unstable, terminal, or contagious conditions that require observation and ongoing treatment; managing intravenous therapy, tube feeding, and vital signs; receiving dialysis, oxygen, and suction administration; managing wounds; and operating power-dependent equipment to sustain life. These individuals require the support of trained medical professionals.

In addition to people with needs in these functional areas, the special needs population includes individuals with service animals or pets. The American Veterinary Medical Association estimates that 58% of all U.S. households have pets. The American Society for the Prevention of Cruelty to Animals notes that more than 30% of the people who did not evacuate during Hurricane Katrina chose to remain with their animals.

The Department of Health and Human Services (HHS) provides a planning resource to identify vulnerable populations in each community. The HHS emPOWER Map provides a map to assist responders in emergency preparedness, response, and recovery. The resource is available at the Public Health Emergency HHS emPOWER Map website (http://empowermap.phe.gov/).

During a larger disaster in the community, it is best to not overload the hospital with nonacute patients. Alternative dispositions should be considered based on community emergency response plans and applicable regulations.

Depending on community emergency response plans and applicable regulations, evacuees might be transported by ambulance to a shelter or a special medical needs shelter. Special medical needs shelters are designed to keep displaced noninstitutionalized individuals who need assistance with activities of daily living out of a hospital setting during an emergency.

Special medical needs shelters may provide assistance with oxygen, blood glucose monitoring, basic wound care,

and medication compliance. Higher-acuity patients may be cared for in the out-of-hospital environment based on the capabilities of the local jurisdiction or resources brought in for the response (such as a disaster medical assistance team).

CHECK YOUR KNOWLEDGE

When planning for the evacuation of patients with special needs, EMS providers need to consider all of the following needs *except*:

A. communication.
B. health insurance provider.
C. medical care.
D. supervision.

Patient Tracking

The Health and Social Services Committee of the New Orleans Commission recommended "generating databases with reliable and up-to-date demographic information that can contribute to enhancing hospital planning and decision-making during crisis situations." The need for information with which to plan and respond is relevant both to those communities directly impacted by an event and to those communities serving as a lifeboat in accepting evacuees. These tracking needs are compounded by the fact that many complex evacuations across the United States involved an average of 3.5 moves, most of which were made across state lines.

Health care workers in Houston, Texas, receiving evacuees from areas affected by Hurricane Katrina found that many evacuees coming from the Superdome shelter in New Orleans, Louisiana, and from other shelters arrived with

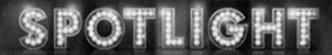

What Should You Take to the Shelter With the Patient?

- Medications
- Oxygen supply
- Nasal cannula and tubing
- Home nebulizer machine
- Walker or other ambulatory aids
- Hearing aids and glasses
- Medical records
- Service animal
- Based on local practice, nonservice animals

pressing medical needs such as chronic illnesses, prescription refills for missing medications, replacement of eyeglasses, basic dental needs, and psychiatric services.

Methods that EMS providers can use to preserve essential medical information with each evacuee includes transporting printed medical records with the patient or using electronic medical records via a regional health information organization. Patients should be tracked through an emergency operations center, a multiple agency coordination center, or a health care evacuation center.

CHECK YOUR KNOWLEDGE

Evacuee medical records can be tracked through a(n):

A. multiple agency coordination center.
B. health care evacuation center.
C. emergency operations center.
D. All of the above.

SUMMARY

- A disaster can be broken down into five phases: the quiescence or interdisaster phase, the prodrome or warning phase, the impact phase, the response phase, and the recovery and reconstruction phase.
- Emergency management planning has four phases: mitigation, planning, response, and recovery. Some authorities may include a fifth phase: prevention.
- The purpose of evacuations is to save and protect the lives of people exposed to actual or imminent danger through their timely and rapid movement to safer locations and places of shelter. With the threat and impact of natural disasters such as severe storms, floods, earthquakes, and wild fires, hundreds to millions of people may need to move within a very short period.
- Sheltering-in-place may become the preferred option to avoid exposure to outside environmental hazards, such as radiologic or airborne contaminants. Building and safety personnel, homeowners, and residents should have contingencies to move to and/or create safe rooms and designated safe areas if sheltering-in-place is recommended.
- Members of a special needs population have needs before, during, and after an incident in the functional areas of maintaining independence, communication, transportation, supervision, and medical care. Individuals with service animals or pets are also considered members of a special needs population.
- Essential medical information needs to be tracked and preserved with each evacuee either by transporting printed medical records with the patient or by using electronic medical records via a regional health information organization.

REFERENCES AND ADDITIONAL RESOURCES

Abt Associates Inc. (2006, May). *Estimating loss of life from hurricane-related flooding in the greater New Orleans area: Health effects of Hurricane Katrina.* Cambridge, MA: Abt Associates.

Agency for Healthcare Research and Quality. (January, 2009). *Recommendations for a national mass patient and evacuee movement, regulating, and tracking system.* Rockville, MD: Author. Retrieved from https://www.hsdl .org/?view&did=38699

Alexander, D. (2002). *Principles of emergency planning and management.* Oxford, United Kingdom: Oxford University Press.

Alliance. (2011, September 27). *Mass evacuation process guide: Los Angeles operational area.* Retrieved from http://catastrophicplanning.org/products/LAOA_Mass_Evacuation_Guide_SEP2011.pdf

Bring New Orleans Back Commission. (2006). *Report: Infrastructure committee; Levees and flood protection, January 18, 2006.* Health and Social Services Committee of the New Orleans Commission. Retrieved from http://www.columbia.edu/itc/journalism/cases/katrina/city_of_new_orleans_bnobc.html

CCCM Steering Committee. (2015). *The mend guide: Comprehensive guide for planning mass evacuations in natural disasters. Pilot document.* Camp Coordination and Camp Management (CCCM) Cluster. Retrieved from http://www.globalcccmcluster.org/system/files/publications/MEND_download.pdf

Dosa, D., Hyer, K., Thomas, K., Swaminathan, S., Feng, Z., Brown, L., and Mor, V. (2012). To evacuate or shelter in place: Implications of universal hurricane evacuation policies on nursing home residents. *Journal of the American Medical Directors Association, 13*(2). doi:10.1016/j.jamda.2011.07.011

Dostal, P. J. (2015). Vulnerability of urban homebound older adults in disasters: A survey of evacuation preparedness. *Disaster Medicine and Public Health Preparedness, 9*(03), 301–306. doi:10.1017/dmp.2015.50

Federal Highway Administration. (2009, April). *Evacuating populations with special needs: Routes to effective evacuation planning primer series.* Washington, DC: U.S. Department of Transportation. Retrieved from https://www.hsdl.org/?view&did=35645

Furin, M. A., and Brenner, B. E. (2016). Disaster planning. MedScape. WebMD. Retrieved from http://emedicine.medscape.com/article/765495-overview#a1

Internal Displacement Monitoring Centre. (2013, May 13). *Global estimates 2012: People displaced by disasters.* Retrieved from http://www.internal-displacement.org/publications/2013/global-estimates-2012-people-displaced-by-disasters

Noji, E. K., and Sivertson, K. T. (1987). Injury prevention in natural disasters: A theoretical framework. *Disasters, 11*, 290.

Waugh, W. L., Jr. (2007). Local emergency management in the post-9/11 world. In W. L. Waugh, Jr., and K. T. Tierney (Eds.), *Emergency management: Principles and practice for local government* (2nd ed.). Washington, DC: ICMA Press.

4 Triage

OBJECTIVES

After studying this chapter, you will be able to:

- Discuss the difference between primary and secondary triage.

- Explain how triage is impacted when resources are limited.

- Identify the limitations to current triage algorithms.

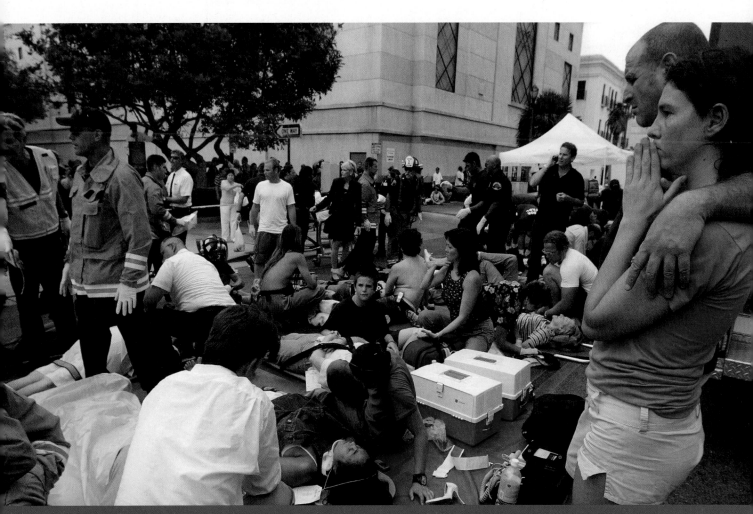

© Carlos Chavez/Los Angeles Times/Getty.

Triage and All Hazards Disasters

Triage is the process prehospital providers use to sort patients and establish a priority process for treatment and transport. When there are sufficient resources and no incident hazards or challenges, triage identifies the patients with the most life-threatening injuries as being the first to receive care and the first to be transported. A **mass-casualty incident (MCI)** is any incident in which emergency medical services resources are overwhelmed by the number and severity of casualties.

Primary Triage

The first arriving EMS providers at an MCI need to assess the scope of the incident. During **primary triage**, the number of casualties, the severity of their condition, and the additional or specialized resources needed are determined using the **sort, assess, lifesaving interventions, treatment/ triage (SALT)** assessment. The SALT system starts with a global sorting process that involves asking victims to walk

or wave (follow commands). Those who do not respond are assessed for life threats, with very limited lifesaving interventions and a fast assessment performed.

Patients are categorized into immediate, delayed, minimal, expectant, or dead (**FIGURE 4-1**). At the completion of primary triage, the incident commander has a count of the number of casualties, an assessment of their severity status, and the need for special resources.

Secondary Triage

Secondary triage is performed when the patients arrive at the treatment or holding area. More extensive assessment is provided, usually using the simple triage and rapid treatment (START) triage scheme, validating or updating the severity of the patient. The priority of care for each person, designated at the scene by color (red for immediate, yellow for delayed, and green for minimal), determines the treatment area to which each patient is taken. More extensive lifesaving interventions may be performed, but the primary goal is to quickly move patients to an appropriate medical care facility (**FIGURE 4-2**).

mass-casualty incident (MCI) Any incident in which emergency medical services resources, such as personnel and equipment, are overwhelmed by the number and severity of casualties.

primary triage The process by which initial prehospital providers assess the scope of the incident, including the number of casualties, the severity of their condition, and the additional or specialized resources needed.

sort, assess, lifesaving interventions, treatment/ triage (SALT) A triage system that is a national guideline for handling MCIs.

secondary triage A more detailed assessment performed when the patient arrives at the treatment/ transport area.

CHECK YOUR KNOWLEDGE

An abdominal evisceration wound would be covered and stabilized:

A. during primary triage.
B. during secondary triage.
C. during transport.
D. after arrival at a medical center.

Limitations of Triage Systems

Triage dates back to the early 1800s, when a surgeon in Napoleon's army, Dominique Jean Larrey, created a system of categorizing war casualties and treating the various types of injuries

SPOTLIGHT

30-Second SALT Triage and Lifesaving Interventions

• Control major hemorrhage.
• Open airway. Consider two rescue breaths if the victim is a child.

• Provide chest decompression.
• Administer auto-injector antidotes.

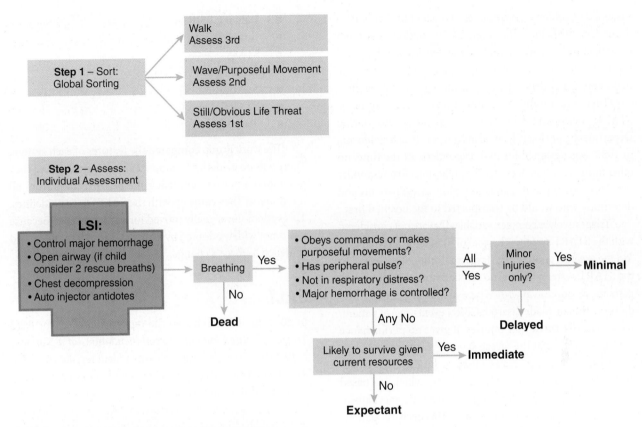

Figure 4-1 SALT mass-casualty triage algorithm.

Reproduced from Federal Interagency Committee on EMS (2014) *National Implementation Of the Model Uniform Core Criteria for Mass Casualty Incident Triage.* Washington DC: U. S. Department of Transportation. Appendix A.

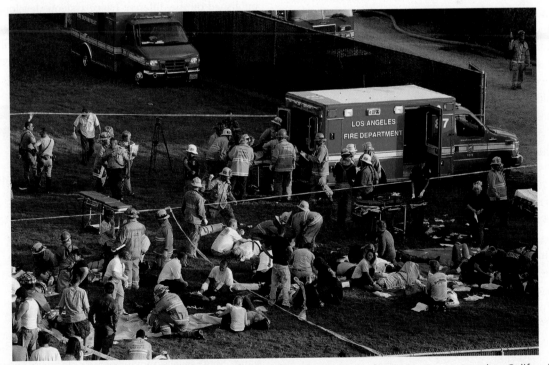

Figure 4-2 The setup of a treatment and transport area after the 2008 train collision in Los Angeles, California. There were 135 injuries and 25 fatalities.

© Brian Vander Brug/Brian Vander Brug/Getty.

sustained by soldiers. Triage has grown out of the battlefields to modern medicine. It has been used to decide what types of ambulances should respond to emergencies, which patient should be transported first from the prehospital setting, and, in the emergency department, to define who gets treated first.

There are a number of limitations to triage systems. START, developed by the Newport Beach Fire and Marine Department and Hoag Hospital in Newport Beach California in 1983, was designed for first responders. At the time, no other formalized system existed for prehospital first responder use. This system was designed to rapidly assess patients and determine who would be transported to the hospital first.

Triage involves complex variables that are not considered with the START system. The goal of managing an MCI is to "do the greatest good for the largest number of patients." In the START system, there is no consideration for number of patients, resource availability, type of incident (e.g., natural disaster, human-made disaster, CBRN event), age of patient, scene hazards, threats, or injuries. It gives no performance measures as to what the "greatest good" really means.

In 1986, The American College of Surgeons (ACS) developed the Field Triage Decision Scheme, which was based on four decision steps: physiological, anatomic, mechanism of injury, and special considerations. This decision scheme was established for prehospital providers to apply a more scientific approach in selecting the hospital to which the patients should be transported. Trauma centers were increasing in popularity, and a way to identify who would benefit most from the transport to the trauma center was developed.

A modification was made to START in 1996. Secondary assessment of victim endpoint (SAVE) was developed based on a catastrophic disaster model that would overwhelm local resources and would allow responders to direct limited resources to casualties who could benefit the most from immediate care. SAVE was studied and compared patients with types of injuries and survivability based on the trauma statistics available in 1996. This modification was not widely taught to prehospital providers, nor is it used in most systems that use START.

In 2004, the Centers for Disease Control and Prevention (CDC) sponsored the Mass-Casualty Triage Project in an effort to lead the development of national guidelines for mass-casualty triage. The Terrorism Injuries: Information Dissemination and Exchange Project was created to review available evidence on triage and develop a national standard for mass-causality triage. A work group was established with a number of organizational stakeholders, from physician groups to EMS providers. They reviewed a number of triage systems:

- CareFlight
- French Red Plan or ORSEC
- Glasgow Coma Scale
- Homebush
- Italian CESIRA
- JumpSTART (pediatric)
- MASS
- Military/NATO Triage
- Sacco
- START
- Triage Sieve

The work group compared the features of each system. There was no evidence to support any one system, and they developed a new system using the best practices from all the systems. They came up with the SALT triage guidelines. This system never really moved forward, however, because it was not widely adopted by all the stakeholders and lacked evidence to force a change.

SALT

In 2012, the CDC released the report *Guidelines for Field Triage of Injured Patients: Recommendations of a National Expert Panel on Field Triage*. This document revisited the 1986 ACS Field Triage Decision Scheme and reviewed the latest data posted since the last work group meetings in 2006. The SALT triage scheme was intended to develop a methodology that would be the basis for a national triage system for MCIs following the science- and consensus-based Model Uniform Core Criteria (MUCC).

Numerous studies have been conducted and articles published on the different triage systems developed since START in 1983; however, no empirical evidence has proven that one system is the best. Because communities will choose what is best for their first responders, no consensus has been reached regarding creating one national triage system.

 CHECK YOUR KNOWLEDGE

Which triage system considers issues of mass-casualty triage following the Model Uniform Core Criteria?

A. JumpSTART
B. ORSEC
C. SALT
D. Triage Sieve

Working an MCI

Triage begins where you land on the scene, or "where you stand." Some suggest moving out in a clockwise fashion or in an ever-increasing concentric circle beginning with the first patient you encounter, then the next, and so on. It is important to understand that you should not seek out the most critical patient; if you do so, you will be moving in an uncoordinated manner and will take longer finding that person than if you were to triage each patient as you come to him or her.

> ## Operations
>
> Remember, triage is a quick assessment. Determine criticality, then move to the next patient.

Which Priority 1 (Red Tag) Patient Goes First?

Which red tag patient needs the most definitive care? Which patient's life will be saved with immediate medical care? At the Boston Marathon bombings, immediate tourniquets applied by bystanders out of makeshift materials saved patients' lives.

A study on the effectiveness of START and START-like methodology identified limitations:

1. The goal of "doing the greatest good for the greatest number" is imprecise. There is no measure of outcome, and results cannot be replicated.

2. There is no consideration of resource availability. Immediates are transported first irrespective of the resources available. As a result, the START triage strategy for a 20-victim incident, for example, is the same whether there are 2 ambulances or 10.

3. There is no differentiation between victim severities within categories, although the severities within immediates and delayeds can vary widely. Also, there can be significant severity overlap between immediates and delayeds.

4. Victim survival probability is not considered explicitly when triaging victims.

5. There is no consideration for or differentiation among trauma types. These limitations lead to subjective and extremely inconsistent triaging.

Essential Patient Information

EMS providers need to start an information path for every patient treated, using a multi-casualty recorder sheet (**FIGURE 4-3**). Data elements to consider recording include the following:

- Patient's name
- Patient's admission date

MULTI-CASUALTY RECORDER WORKSHEET

Ambulance Company	Ambulance ID Number	Patient Triage Tag Number	Patient Status	Hospital Destination	Off Scene Time
			(I) (D) (M)		___ : ___
			(I) (D) (M)		___ : ___
			(I) (D) (M)		___ : ___
			(I) (D) (M)		___ : ___
			(I) (D) (M)		___ : ___
			(I) (D) (M)		___ : ___
			(I) (D) (M)		___ : ___
			(I) (D) (M)		___ : ___
			(I) (D) (M)		___ : ___
			(I) (D) (M)		___ : ___
			(I) (D) (M)		___ : ___
			(I) (D) (M)		___ : ___

Figure 4-3 Detail of a multi-casualty recorder sheet.

Reproduced from Firescope ICS-MC-306 accessed January 19, 2017 from www.firescope.org/ics-multi-casual/forms/ICS-MC-306.pdf. The National Fire Academy would like to thank FIRESCOPE for the use of the Field Operations Guide (ICS 420-1) as a template for this document.

- Patient identification number
- Mode of transportation (ambulance, helicopter, private vehicle)
- Receiving facility/transfer destination
- Attending physician
- Receiving physician (if available)

An all hazards disaster response requires that EMS providers obtain the big picture of triage needs as soon as possible and get adequate human, medical, and support resources to the event. This scene size-up and organization of EMS response will provide the best outcomes for the largest number of people impacted by the event.

CHECK YOUR KNOWLEDGE

As the first arriving EMS unit at an explosion, the most important task on arrival is to:

A. find and transport the most severely injured patient to a burn center.
B. establish the treatment area.
C. contact medical control.
D. determine the total number of injured patients and their severity.

SUMMARY

- Triage is the process prehospital providers use to sort patients and establish a priority process for treatment and transport. When there are sufficient resources and no incident hazards or challenges, triage identifies the patients with the most life-threatening injuries as being the first to receive care and the first to be transported.
- Numerous studies have been conducted and articles published on the different triage systems developed since START in 1983; however, no empirical evidence has proven that one system is the best. Because communities will choose what is best for their first responders, no consensus has been reached regarding creating one national triage system.
- Triage begins where you land on the scene, or "where you stand." Some suggest moving out in a clockwise fashion or in an ever-increasing concentric circle beginning with the first patient encountered, then the next, and so on.

REFERENCES AND ADDITIONAL RESOURCES

Benson, M., Koenig, K. L., and Schultz, C. H. (1996). Disaster triage: START, then SAVE—a new method of dynamic triage for victims of a catastrophic earthquake. *Prehospital and Disaster Medicine, 11*(2), 117–124.

Centers for Disease Control and Prevention. (2012). Guidelines for field triage of injured patients: Recommendations of a national expert panel on field triage, 2011. *Morbidity and Mortality Weekly Report, 61*(1). Retrieved from https://www.facs.org/~/media/files/quality%20programs/trauma/vrc%20resources/6_guidelines%20field%20triage%202011.ashx

Federal Interagency Committee on EMS. (2014). *National implementation of the Model Uniform Core Criteria for Mass Casualty Incident Triage*. Washington, DC: U.S. Department of Transportation. Retrieved from http://www.nhtsa.gov/staticfiles/nti/pdf/811891-Model_UCC_for_Mass_Casualty_Incident_Triage.pdf

Gourgiotis, S. (2009). Baron Dominique-Jean Larrey: Founder of military surgery and trauma care. *Hektoen International Journal*. Retrieved from http://www.hekint.org/index.php/2013-09-27-12-57-30?id=2131

Institute of Medicine. (2011). *Preparedness and response to a rural mass casualty incident: Workshop summary*. Washington, DC: National Academies Press. Retrieved from https://www.ems.gov/pdf/2011/July2011 /9-Preparedness_Response.to.Rural.MCI.IOM2011.pdf

Lerner, E. B., Schwartz, R. B., Coule, P. L., Weinstein, E. S., Cone, D. C., Hunt, R. C., . . . O'Connor, R. E. (2008, September). Mass casualty triage: An evaluation of the data and development of a proposed national guideline. *Disaster Medicine and Public Health Preparedness, 2*(Suppl 1), S25–S34.

Navin, M., and Sacco, W. (2010). Operational comparison of the simple triage and rapid treatment method and the Sacco triage method in mass casualty exercises. *Journal of Trauma: Injury Infection and Critical Care, 69*(1). Retrieved from http://journals.lww.com/jtrauma/Abstract/2010/07000/Operational_Comparison_of_the _Simple_Triage_and.34.aspx

Sacco, W., Navin, D. M., Waddell, R. K., 2nd, Fiedler, K. E., Long, W. B., and Buckman, R. F., Jr. (2007). A new resource-constrained triage method applied to victims of penetrating injury. *The Journal of Trauma: Injury, Infection and Critical Care, 63*(2), 316–325.

Sasser, S. M., Hunt, R. C., Faul, M., Sugerman, D., Pearson, W. S., Dulski, T., and Galli, R. L. (2009). Guidelines for field triage of injured patients recommendations of national expert panel on field triage. *Morbidity and Mortality Weekly Report, 61*. Retrieved from https://www.cdc.gov/mmwr/preview/mmwrhtml/rr5801a1 .htm#fig1

Schenk, J. D., Goldstein, S., Braun, J., Werner, A., Buccellato, F., Asaeda, G., and Prezant, D. J. (2006). Triage accuracy at a multiple casualty incident disaster drill: The Emergency Medical Service, Fire Department of New York City experience. *Journal of Burn Care and Research, 27*(5), 570–575.

U.S. Department of Health and Human Services. (2016). *Triage guidelines.* Radiation Emergency Medical Management. Retrieved from https://www.remm.nlm.gov/radtriage.htm

U.S. Fire Administration. (2012, June). *Operational templates and guidance for EMS mass incident deployment*. Washington, DC: Federal Emergency Management Administration. Retrieved from https://www.usfa.fema .gov/downloads/pdf/publications/templates_guidance_ems_mass_incident_deployment.pdf

U.S. Fire Administration. (2013, September). *Fire/emergency medical services department operational considerations and guide for active shooter and mass casualty incidents*. Washington, DC: Federal Emergency Management Administration. Retrieved from https://www.usfa.fema.gov/downloads/pdf/publications/active _shooter_guide.pdf

CRITICAL THINKING SKILL STATION

Triage Exercise

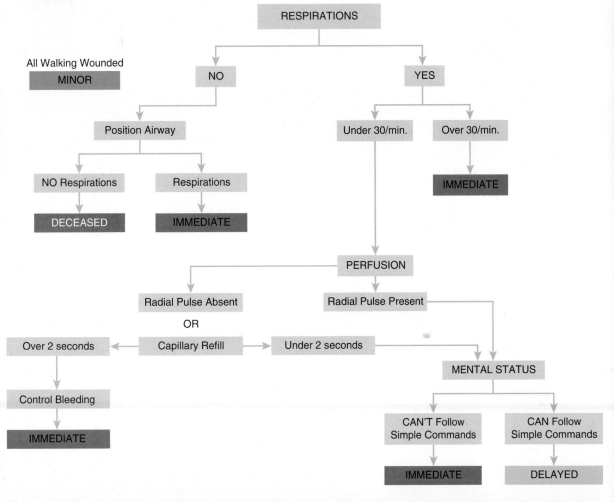

Patient	Respirations	Perfusion	Mental Status	Triage Tag Color
1				
2				
3				
4				
5				

Based on the video shown, use this worksheet to determine each color triage tag that should be placed on the patient.

Transportation Incidents

OBJECTIVES

After studying this chapter, you will be able to:

- Discuss how to adequately utilize scarce resources during the initial stages of an incident.

- List common factors that identify special needs of populations and potential challenges.

- Explain how shifting the focus of patient care from individual outcomes to population outcomes changes patient management in resource-scarce environments.

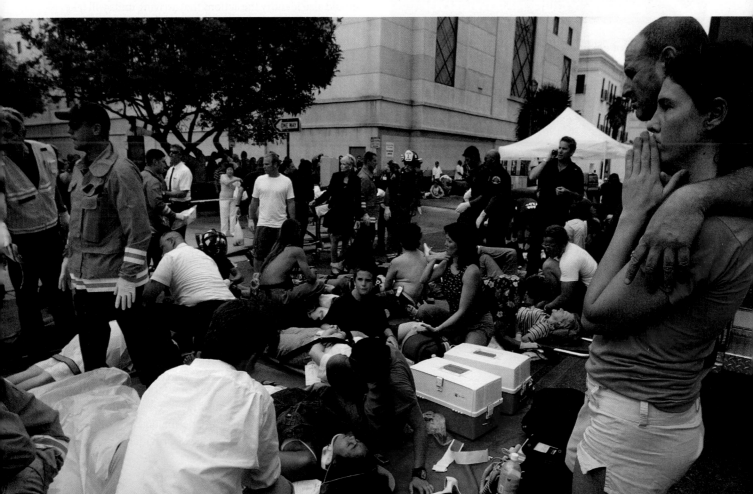

Role of Emergency Medical Dispatchers

Emergency medical dispatchers (EMDs) are the first EMS providers involved in a transportation event. They send out the nearest responders while gathering additional details on the event. For the scenario in this chapter, a bus carrying people with special needs is involved in the collision. The EMD will attempt to determine what type of special needs exist and what additional resources are required. Special needs may involve individuals with service animals and people with mental or physical disabilities. Patients may be in wheelchairs and on ventilators.

One regional resource in many communities is a major emergency response vehicle or medical ambulance bus. The 42-foot unit comes equipped with stretchers to accommodate 24 patients and medical personnel for transport, patient monitoring equipment, metered oxygen, electrical capacity to supply power for necessary medical equipment, and rehabilitation supplies, all in a climate-controlled area (**FIGURE 5-1**).

CHECK YOUR KNOWLEDGE

The role of emergency medical dispatchers in a major incident include all the following *except*:

A. initiating the incident action plan.
B. sending out the nearest responders.
C. continuing to gather additional information on the event.
D. determining what type of special needs exist.

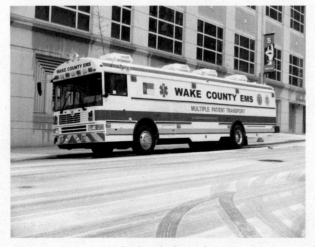

Figure 5-1 A medical ambulance bus.
© Mike Legeros. Used with permission.

Scene Size-up

The first arriving EMS providers are expected to assume command of the incident. The initial incident commander (IC) remains in charge of the incident until command is transferred or the situation is stabilized and terminated. If the incident expands, a higher ranking officer is likely to arrive and assume command, at which point the initial IC's role changes.

Command must be established, and the incident command system (ICS) must be used at every event. For incidents requiring two or more responding resources, the initial EMS responder on the scene must establish command and initiate an incident management structure that is appropriate for the incident. Check with your local jurisdictions to determine who is designated as the agency responsible for a unified command for a major event on an interstate highway.

Activating the command process includes providing an initial radio report and announcing that command has been established. This report should provide an accurate description of the situation for units that are still en route. It should also identify the actions that arriving units will take. In this report, the initial IC should include the following information:

- Identification of the unit arriving at the scene
- A brief description of the incident situation, such as magnitude of a multiple-vehicle collision
- Obvious conditions, such as a working fire, multiple patients, a hazardous materials spill, or a dangerous situation, such as a man with a gun
- A brief description of the action to be taken (e.g., "Ambulance 611 is starting primary triage.")
- Any obvious safety concerns
- Assumption, identification, and location of command
- Request for additional resources (or release of resources), if required

Levels of Command

The ICS includes three levels of command, with a set of responsibilities being assigned to each level. At small-scale incidents or in the early stages of a larger incident, one EMS provider may cover all three levels simultaneously. When the incident expands, the management responsibilities are subdivided. An EMS provider may have a role at any level.

SPOTLIGHT

M-E-T-H-A-N-E Method of Scene Size-up

- **M**ass-casualty incident declared by IC
- **E**xact location
- **T**ype of incident—traffic accident, explosion

- **H**azards present—weather conditions, hazardous materials
- **A**ccess and egress—assessment of primary and secondary routes to scene

- **N**umber of casualties and severity—how many immediate, delayed, minimal, and dead
- **E**mergency services required— hazardous materials, technical rescue, heating/cooling stations

The overall direction and goals are set at the **strategic level**. The IC always functions at the strategic level. **Tactical-level** objectives define the actions that are necessary to achieve the strategic goals. A tactical-level supervisor would manage a group of resources to accomplish the tactical objective. In medium- to large-scale incidents, the tactical-level components would be called **divisions**, **groups**, or units, and each of these components could include several ambulances from different organizations. All ambulances would report to the tactical-level supervisor. Tactical assignments are usually defined by a geographic area (e.g., one part of a building) or a functional responsibility (e.g., extrication), or sometimes by a combination of the two (e.g., occupant removal in a specific section of the building).

In large incidents, another level of management may be added to maintain a reasonable span of control. Branches are established to group tactical components. An officer assigned to a branch would oversee some combination of divisions, groups, or units.

Task-level assignments are the actions required to achieve the tactical objectives. The physical work is accomplished at this level. Individual units or teams of responders perform task-level activities, such as treating red tag patients, transporting patients, or providing responder rehabilitation services.

The initial IC identifies the triage, treatment, and transport sectors of the incident and requests adequate resources to cover all three areas. Traffic flow and access will be an issue.

 CHECK YOUR KNOWLEDGE

EMS providers working on patients in the treatment area are performing work at the _____ level.

A. strategic
B. tactical
C. strike force
D. task

strategic level The command level that entails the overall direction and goals of the incident.

tactical level The command level in which objectives must be achieved to meet the strategic goals. The tactical-level supervisor or officer is responsible for completing assigned objectives.

division A supervisory level established to divide an incident into geographic areas of operations.

group A supervisory level established to divide the incident into functional areas of operations.

task level The command level in which specific tasks are assigned to units or teams; these tasks are geared toward meeting tactical-level requirements.

Ambulance Strike Team

EMS providers may be part of an **ambulance strike team**. The mission of the ambulance strike team is to provide supplemental medical transportation during large-scale patient movements or other special circumstances. A strike team will be assembled at the request of the IC, based on local jurisdiction practice or procedure. Each ambulance strike team is five ambulances under the direction of an ambulance strike team leader (ASTL) in a separate vehicle. The six vehicles in the strike team (five ambulances plus the ASTL vehicle) must have common communications (**FIGURE 5-2**).

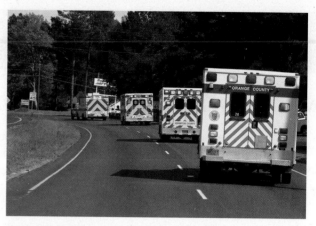

Figure 5-2 An ambulance strike team.
© Mike Legeros. Used with permission.

Scene Safety

Transportation incidents increase the risk to EMS providers due to an exponential rise in the impact of smartphones on vehicle collisions. In 2014, a total of 3,179 people were killed and 431,000 were injured in motor vehicle crashes involving distracted drivers.

To stay safe on the scene of a vehicle collision, EMS responders should wear the following personal protective equipment:

- Turnout gear
- Safety gloves
- Helmet
- Safety goggles
- A vest approved by the American National Standards Institute

CHECK YOUR KNOWLEDGE

Appropriate safety outerwear while operating at a transportation incident must:

A. identify your organization.
B. be approved by the American National Standards Institute.
C. show two contrasting colors.
D. have retro-reflective material on more than 40% of the surface area.

ambulance strike team An ICS resource consisting of five ambulances and a supervisor or support vehicle operating under a shared communication system.

Patients With Special Needs

Patients with special needs may present a wide variety of challenges, requiring the responder to modify communications, assessments, treatment, and transport actions. Special needs may include a service animal or mobility chair. Patients may use a ventilator, feeding tube, central line, or colostomy bag. Patients may have seeing or hearing impairments. Patients may also have mental or physical disabilities. Each patient will present a specific set of needs. The staff or family members caring for individuals with special needs will be an important resource when assessing these patients.

Consider patients with special needs to be priority patients, to be moved to an appropriate medical destination as soon as the life-threatening immediate or red tag patients are transported. Additional EMS providers may be required during transport due to the complexity or severity of the person's condition.

CHECK YOUR KNOWLEDGE

When setting transport priorities, patients with special needs should be transported:

A. first.
B. after red tags.
C. after yellow tags.
D. after green tags.

SUMMARY

- Emergency medical dispatchers (EMDs) are the first EMS providers involved in a transportation event, sending out the nearest responders while gathering additional details on the event.
- The first arriving EMS providers are expected to assume command of the incident, providing an initial radio report and announcing that command has been established. This report should provide an accurate description of the situation for units that are still en route and should identify the actions that arriving units will take.
- EMS providers may be part of an ambulance strike team, providing supplemental medical transportation during large-scale patient movements or other special circumstances. Each ambulance strike team contains five ambulances under the direction of an ambulance strike team leader in a separate vehicle.
- Patients with special needs may present a wide variety of challenges, requiring the EMS provider to modify communications, assessments, treatment, and transport actions. Patients with special needs should be considered priority patients, to be moved to an appropriate medical destination as soon as any life-threatening immediate or red tag patients are transported.

REFERENCES AND ADDITIONAL RESOURCES

Division of Public Health. (n.d.). *Children with special health care needs: Provider manual*. Atlanta, GA: Georgia Department of Public Health. Retrieved from https://dph.georgia.gov/sites/dph.georgia.gov/files/cwshcnprovidermanual.04.pdf

Emergency Medical Task Force. (2012). *Ambulance strike team standard operating guidelines*. Texas Department of Health. Retrieved from http://www.tdms.org/ContentHandler.ashx?ID=12745

Federal Emergency Management Agency. (2011). *National Incident Management System: Training program*. Washington, DC: U.S. Department of Homeland Security. Retrieved from https://training.fema.gov/emiweb/is/icsresource/assets/nims_training_program.pdf

Federal Emergency Management Agency. (2013). *National response framework* (2nd ed.). Washington, DC: U.S. Department of Homeland Security. Retrieved from https://www.fema.gov/media-library-data/20130726-1914-25045-1246/final_national_response_framework_20130501.pdf

Federal Highway Administration. (2009). *Evacuating populations with special needs: Route to effective evacuation planning primer series*. Washington, DC: U.S. Department of Transportation. Retrieved from http://www.ops.fhwa.dot.gov/publications/fhwahop09022/fhwahop09022.pdf

NC EMSC Advisory Committee. (2009.) Recommended EMS guidelines for children and youth with special health care needs (CYSHCN). Office of Emergency Medical Services. Retrieved from https://www.ncems.org/pdf/CYSHCNPrehospitalGuidelinesJuly2009.pdf

Northern Virginia Operations Board. (2013, May). *EMS multiple casualty incident manual* (2nd ed.). Fairfax, VA: Fire and Rescue Departments of Northern Virginia. Retrieved from http://fcfra.camp9.org/Resources/Documents/FOG/MCI%20Manual%20(NOVA).pdf

Texas Engineering Extension Service. (2010). *Ambulance strike team/medical task force (AST/MTF) leader. Participant manual*. Emergency Services Training Institute. Retrieved from http://www.cbrac.org/uploads/CBRAC/EMTFASTLClassCC.pdf

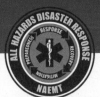

CRITICAL THINKING SKILL STATION

LCAN Report

Location

- Street
- Highway
- Residence
- Multifamily dwelling
- Commercial building

Conditions

- Where you are
- Any obstacles
- Smoke
- Visibility
- Entrapped patients
- Container type
- Number of patients

Actions

- Establishing command
- Beginning triage
- Evacuating the area

Needs

- Reinforcements
  – Who, specifically?
- Relief
- Tools or equipment
- Cover other areas
- More ambulances

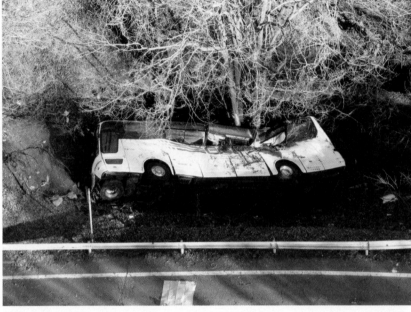

© Jun Yasukawa/The Yomiuri Shimbun/AP Photo

Giving an on-scene report over the radio is critical to the first few minutes of any incident. It will help dispatch as well as other responding units get a picture of what the first on-scene unit is facing. It is an opportunity for the first unit to relay vital information about where the incident is, what type of problems are being faced, what that unit is doing in the next several minutes, and what type of help they need.

The initial incident action plan (IAP) is developed by the first unit (this takes place quickly) based on the basic information that is initially observed.

Based on what you see in the picture above, develop an LCAN report. With one person from the group acting as the team leader, have the team members write down what the leader says, then have the leader or someone the leader assigns make a radio report to the class.

L _____

C _____

A _____

N _____

6 Infectious Disease

OBJECTIVES

After studying this chapter, you will be able to:

- Identify infectious agents that an emergency medical services (EMS) provider may encounter.

- Describe sources of credible information for EMS providers during an infectious disease event.

- Explain actions to take while responding to an infectious disease event.

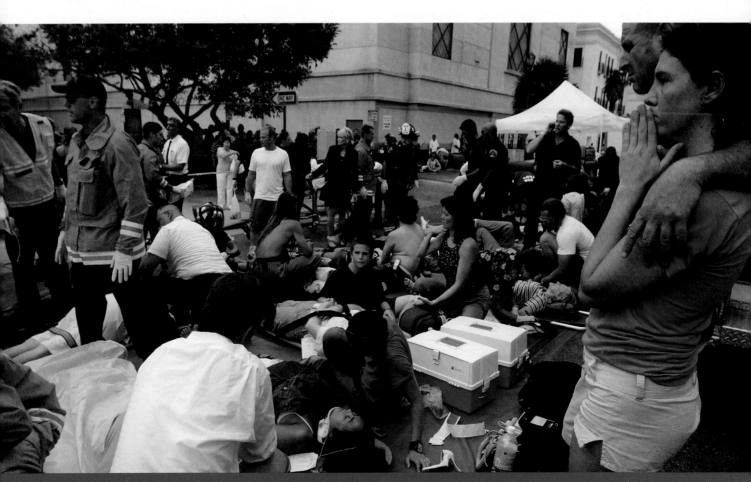

© Carlos Chavez/Los Angeles Times/Getty.

Infectious and Communicable Diseases

Infectious diseases are illnesses caused by pathogenic organisms such as bacteria, viruses, fungi, and parasites. Most infectious diseases, such as the common cold, are not life threatening. **Communicable diseases** are a subset of infectious diseases that can be transmitted from person to person. Communicable diseases pose a threat to EMS providers.

Infectious diseases are spread from person to person in four ways:

1. **Contact transmission.** Contact can be direct or indirect. An example of direct contact is touching a patient. Venereal diseases, such as syphilis and gonorrhea, are spread through direct contact. A contaminated needlestick is another example. Indirect contact occurs by touching or handling an infected object or coming into contact with a person contaminated with pathogens from a person or the person's secretions.

2. **Droplet transmission.** Droplets from an infected person are spread through close person-to-person contact, such as kissing, hugging, sharing eating or drinking utensils, or talking within a 3-foot (0.9-m) radius. Performing mouth-to-mouth ventilation without a barrier is an example of droplet transmission for EMS providers.

3. **Airborne transmission.** A vapor of infectious particles is suspended in the air for long periods of time. Tuberculosis is an example of an infectious communicable disease spread through airborne transmission. Patients with compromised immune systems and those living or working in densely populated areas are most at risk from airborne transmission.

4. **Vector transmission.** *Vector* refers to an organism that carries a pathogen to another organism. The vector may harbor a pathogen that is harmless to itself but harmful to humans; by coming into

contact with humans, it may spread that pathogen, causing disease in humans. A bite from a mosquito infected with the West Nile virus is an example of a vector transmission.

Infection control centers on early recognition through proficient assessment. Responders must strike a balance between caring for patients and limiting the spread of infectious agents to others, including themselves. They must always consider the impact of the disease process. The risk of transmission can be limited through these precautions:

- Receive immunizations and vaccinations.
- Use personal protective equipment consistent with the signs and symptoms of infectious disease.
- Pursue postexposure medical reporting and follow-up.
- Gain a broad comprehension of disease progression and management of infected patients.

CHECK YOUR KNOWLEDGE

A patient with an infectious respiratory disease sneezes in the face of a responder. This is an example of _____ transmission.

A. vector
B. airborne
C. droplet
D. contact

Infectious Agents

This section overviews four types of common infectious agents. Because the terms *communicable* and *infectious* are often used interchangeably, it is important to note that while all of the agents that follow can infect humans, not all are communicable; that is, not all the diseases discussed are transmitted from person to person.

Bacteria

Bacteria are single-celled microorganisms that live in water, inside the human body, in organic matter, and on inorganic surfaces (fomites). Antibodies are effective agents against most bacterial infections. Aerobic bacteria, such as those that cause tuberculosis and plague, can survive only in the presence of oxygen. Anaerobic bacteria, such as *Clostridium* strains, which cause botulism and tetanus, carry out their cellular functions without oxygen.

infectious disease An illness caused by pathogenic organisms such as bacteria, viruses, fungi, and parasites. Most infectious diseases, such as the common cold, are not life threatening.

communicable disease Any infectious disease transmitted from one person or animal to another.

Viruses

One of the smallest disease agents, viruses must grow and multiply inside the living cells of a host. Viruses are the source of minor illnesses, such as the common cold, as well as grave diseases, including smallpox and acquired immunodeficiency syndrome (AIDS). Antiviral medications and vaccines have been developed to prevent some lethal viral infections or to moderate the severity of symptoms and reduce the length of illness.

Fungi

Fungi are plantlike microorganisms, most of which are not pathogenic. Yeast, mold, mildew, and mushrooms are types of fungi. Fungi impacting human illness include the following:

- **Dermatophytes.** Skin infections such as tinea corporis (also called ringworm).
- *Aspergillus* **spp.** Pulmonary aspergillosis and infections of the external ear, sinuses, and subcutaneous tissue.
- *Blastomyces dermatitidis.* Blastomycosis, which causes skin and subcutaneous abscesses.
- *Histoplasma capsulatum.* Histoplasmosis caused by breathing in spores from bird or bat droppings.
- *Candida* **spp.** Candidal vulvovaginitis (also called yeast infection and vaginal thrush) and oral candidiasis (also called oral thrush).

Parasites

Parasites are a common cause of disease where sanitation is poor. Unlike viruses, parasites are living organisms. Parasites must have a living host that they live on or feed on. The patient may experience topical or systemic irritation or infection. Antihistamines may be prescribed to relieve urticaria (hives). Insecticides, acetylcholinesterase inhibitors, ovicidals, and pediculicides can be effective treatment/prevention of parasite infection.

 CHECK YOUR KNOWLEDGE

_____ are one of the smallest disease agents.

A. Parasites
B. Viruses
C. Bacteria
D. Fungi

Stages of the Infection Process

Exposure to a pathogen does not mean instant infection—only that the pathogen has entered the host. The chance of infection is based on the pathogen dose (the number of organisms present), the **virulence** of the organism, and the susceptibility of the host. Communicable diseases involve four periods: latent, incubation, communicability, and disease. It should be noted that the communicability period can occur at the same time as other periods.

Latent Period

The latent period begins when the pathogen enters the body by evading the host's outermost layer of defense, such as the skin or acidic mucous secretions. During the latent period, the infection is not communicable and the patient exhibits no symptoms. This period may be as short as one day or may last for months or years.

Incubation Period

The incubation period occurs between the latent period and the onset of symptoms. During this period, the pathogen reproduces in the host. The host's immune system responds by producing specific disease antibodies. Seroconversion, when the antibodies reach a detectable level in the blood, may occur. The incubation period varies from hours to years.

Communicability Period

The communicability period runs as long as the pathogen remains in the body and can be spread to other people. This period varies in length and is dependent on the virulence, the number of organisms that are transmitted, the mode of transportation, and the host's resistance. The age and general health status of the patient prior to exposure affect the susceptibility and risk factors of contracting an infectious disease.

Disease Period

This period starts at the end of the incubation period and lasts until the pathogen is destroyed. Duration of this period depends on the specific pathogen. This period may be symptom-free or exhibit obvious symptoms such as a cough or skin lesion.

virulence The power of a microorganism to produce disease.

TABLE 6-1 Components of the Infectious Disease Process		
Stage	**Begins**	**Ends**
Latent period	With invasion	When the agent can be shed
Incubation period	With invasion	When the disease process begins
Communicability period	When the latent period ends	Continues as long as the agent is present and can spread to others
Disease period	Follows incubation period	Variable duration

© National Association of Emergency Medical Technicians.

Some pathogens, such as the human immunodeficiency virus (HIV) and herpes viruses, will remain in the body indefinitely (**TABLE 6-1**).

CHECK YOUR KNOWLEDGE

A patient is contagious during the _____ period of the infectious process.

A. latent
B. incubation
C. disease
D. None of the above

Epidemics and Pandemics

An **epidemic** is a disease outbreak in which many people in a community or region become infected with the same disease. This outbreak can occur when an outside source carries the pathogen to a host community that has not previously encountered the pathogen and therefore has formed no defenses against it; this scenario occurred when an infected traveler brought severe acute respiratory syndrome (SARS) to Ontario, Canada, from Asia in 2003.

epidemic A disease outbreak in which many people in a community or region become infected with the same disease.

pandemic An epidemic that sweeps the planet, reaching all seven continents.

asymptomatic carrier An infected patient who has no knowledge of the infection but is capable of transmitting the disease to others.

It can also occur when a pathogen that is already familiar to a host community mutates and evades the usual immune response or becomes more virulent. Emergence of a new version of an old disease, such as influenza A strains H1N1 and H5N1, could also cause an epidemic.

A **pandemic** is an epidemic that sweeps the planet, reaching all seven continents. For example, the 1918–1919 influenza A pandemic caused 50 million deaths and infected a third of the world's population. If the source of the pandemic is a virulent new pathogen or a mutant form of an older disease, few people will have the antibodies that make them resistant to the disease.

The Chain of Infection

Infection involves a chain of events through which the communicable disease spreads. Microorganisms residing in the body without causing disease are part of the normal flora and are one layer of infection defense. Normal flora creates environmental conditions hostile to pathogens. This state of balance is called homeostasis.

Reservoir/Host

Pathogens may live and reproduce on and within humans, animal hosts, or other organic substances. Once infected, the human host may show signs and symptoms of the illness or may become an asymptomatic carrier. An **asymptomatic carrier** will have no knowledge of the infection but is capable of transmitting the disease to others. The life cycle of a pathogen depends on the age of the host, genetic factors of the host, the temperature of the host environment, and the efficacy of any therapeutic measures once the infection is recognized.

Portal of Exit

A portal of exit is necessary if a pathogenic agent is to leave one host to infect another. Portals include the genitourinary tract, intestinal tract, oral cavity, respiratory tract, and open lesions.

SPOTLIGHT

Could a 1918 Pandemic Appear Today?

Some characteristics of the 1918 pandemic appear unique. Most notably, death rates were 5–20 times higher than expected. Clinically and pathologically, these high death rates appear to be the result of several factors, including a higher proportion of severe and complicated infections of the respiratory tract. Also, the deaths were concentrated in an unusually young age group. Finally, in 1918, three separate recurrences of influenza followed each other with unusual rapidity, resulting in three explosive pandemic waves within a year's time. Scientists must conclude that since it happened once, analogous conditions could lead to an equally devastating pandemic.

Reproduced from Taubenberger, J. K., and Morens, D. M. (2006). 1918 influenza: The mother of all pandemics. *Emerging Infectious Diseases, 12*(1), 15–22.

Transmission

Direct or indirect transmission may occur through the portal of entry and the portal of exit (**FIGURE 6-1**).

Portal of Entry

The portal of entry is where the pathogenic agent enters a new host. The organism may be ingested, inhaled, or injected through the skin, or it may cross a mucous membrane, the placenta, or nonintact skin. The duration of exposure and the quantity of pathogens required to produce infection in the host differ for each pathogen.

Host Susceptibility

For infection to occur, the host must be susceptible to infection by the pathogen. Susceptibility means the host is unhealthy or in a weakened state and its immune system cannot protect the body (**TABLE 6-2**).

 CHECK YOUR KNOWLEDGE

A patient who is an asymptomatic carrier:

A. has disease signs that appear on only one side of the body.
B. has symptoms of the disease but is no longer infectious.
C. has a dormant form of the disease reactivated by a new exposure.
D. is unaware of having the disease but can infect others.

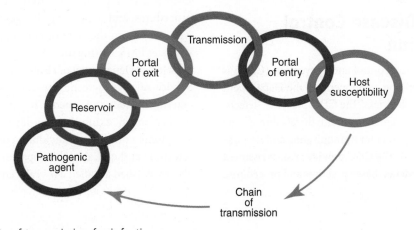

Figure 6-1 Chain of transmission for infection.

© Jones & Bartlett Learning.

TABLE 6-2 Factors That Increase Host Susceptibility to Infection

- *Age.* The very young and the very old are more at risk of contracting an infectious disease.

- *Use of drugs.* Taking immunosuppressive medications, steroids, or other drugs may affect immune response.

- *Malnutrition/obesity.* Poor nutrition weakens the immune system. Obesity is often associated with multiple chronic disease processes and places patients at risk for infection due to a compromised immune system.

- *Chronic disease.* Chronic disease, such as diabetes and heart disease, gradually zaps the body of its ability to defend itself.

- *Shock/trauma.* When a person is in shock or has been injured, body defenses are mobilized to restore organ function and to recover from injury, leaving him or her in a weak position to fight infection.

- *Smoking.* Use of tobacco products has been shown to impair the body's immune system.

© National Association of Emergency Medical Technicians.

Credible Sources of Information

With each incident, EMS providers have obtained more tools and resources to prepare for, respond to, and mitigate the effects of infectious disease pandemics. The 2014 Ebola outbreak in the United States started with an infected patient dying in a Dallas, Texas, hospital. Eventually, 177 people who were directly exposed to the two medical providers infected by "patient zero" required monitoring. Another 285 people were tracked because they were on the same plane as one of the providers. By applying lessons learned from previous disease outbreaks, this incident, which might easily have become a national or even international disaster, was well controlled.

Responders should prepare themselves for the role they may play in the event of a disease outbreak. Credible information is constantly updated and published by subject-matter experts at the federal and international levels.

Centers for Disease Control and Prevention

The Centers for Disease Control and Prevention (CDC) is one of the major operating components of the Department of Health and Human Services. The CDC prevents, detects, and responds to new and emerging health threats through the efforts of the National Center for Immunization and Respiratory Diseases (NCIRD). The CDC provides risk assessment tools and provides evidence-based practices and procedures.

World Health Organization

The World Health Organization (WHO) is a specialized agency of the United Nations that is concerned with international public health. During emergencies, WHO's operational role includes leading and coordinating the health response in support of countries; undertaking risk assessments; identifying priorities and setting strategies; providing critical technical guidance, supplies, and financial resources; and monitoring the health situation. WHO also helps countries to strengthen their national core capacities for emergency risk management to prevent, prepare for, respond to, and recover from emergencies due to any hazard that poses a threat to human health security.

State-Level Departments of Health

EMS is a state-regulated activity, and many directives, procedures, and temporary changes in scope of practice will come from the state or commonwealth agency that regulates EMS. During the U.S. Ebola outbreak of 2014, the New Jersey Department of Health, Communicable Disease Service, reviewed screening results from airport passengers entering the state and issued a "Report Under Investigation" for passengers exhibiting low-level Ebola virus disease symptoms until those individuals completed a follow-up screening at the local health department. The department also established a staffed 24/7 call center.

CHECK YOUR KNOWLEDGE

EMS agencies will change their scope of practice or procedures for handling patients with an infectious disease through directives from the:

A. World Health Organization.
B. Federal Emergency Management Association.
C. Centers for Disease Control and Prevention.
D. relevant state or commonwealth agency that regulates EMS.

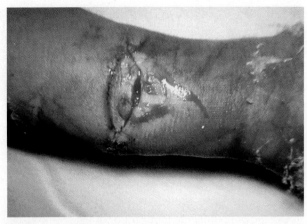
Figure 6-2 Wound botulism.
Courtesy of Centers for Disease Control and Prevention.

Biologic Agents

A **biologic agent** is a pathogen or toxin that may be used as a weapon to spread disease or cause injury to humans. With no dramatic explosion or incident to announce the presence of a biologic agent, there is a longer period of exposure before health officials recognize a pattern of illness. The distribution of anthrax-infected mail in the United States in 2001 is an example of a weaponized biologic agent.

EMS providers need to be vigilant and report any unexpected influx of patients or other atypical patient trends. The Category A pathogens and toxins that can be used as biologic agents include the following:

- **Anthrax**. Acute infectious disease caused by the gram-positive, spore-forming bacterium *Bacillus anthracis*. The most common route of entry is direct skin contact and absorption of spores, which causes a localized red, itchy ulcer. Anthrax spores can also be inhaled. Signs and symptoms appear within 2 weeks of exposure.
- **Botulism**. *Clostridium botulism* produces a nerve toxin that causes paralysis. The route of entry is ingestion of contaminated food and contamination of wounds. Signs and symptoms appear hours or days after exposure (**FIGURE 6-2**).
- **Plague**. *Yersinia pestis* is the bacterium that causes the plague. Normal transmission is through bites of fleas and rodents. Weaponized, the bacterium can be aerosolized, ingested through the lungs, resulting in pneumonic plague. There is a sudden onset of signs and symptoms.

- **Ricin**. *Ricinus communis* is a cytotoxic protein derived from the bean of the castor plant that can be weaponized into an aerosol, powder, or pellet form. Signs and symptoms appear within 8 hours of inhalation, with hypoxia occurring within 36 to 72 hours of exposure.

There are other Category A biologic agents that pose a severe risk without requiring weaponization or special delivery methods. Additional information is available through NAEMT's Advanced Medical Life Support (AMLS) program (**TABLE 6-3**).

CHECK YOUR KNOWLEDGE

_____ is not a Category A biologic agent.

A. *Rickettsia prowazekii*
B. *Ricinus communis*
C. *Yersinia pestis*
D. *Bacillus anthracis*

biologic agent A pathogen or toxin that may be used as a weapon to spread disease or cause injury to humans.

TABLE 6-3 Critical Biologic Agents for Public Health Preparedness

Biologic Agent	Biologic Agent Disease
Category A	
Variola major	Smallpox
Bacillus anthracis	Anthrax
Yersinia pestis	Plague
Clostridium botulinum (botulinum toxins)	Botulism
Francisella tularensis	Tularemia
Filoviruses and arenaviruses (e.g., Ebola, Lassa fever)	Viral hemorrhagic fevers
Category B	
Coxiella burnetii	Q fever
Brucella spp.	Brucellosis
Burkholderia mallei	Glanders
Burkholderia pseudomallei	Melioidosis
Alphaviruses (VEE, EEE, WEE)	Encephalitis
Rickettsia prowazekii	Typhus fever
Toxins (e.g., ricin, staphylococcal enterotoxin B)	Toxic syndromes
Chlamydia psittaci	Psittacosis
Food safety threats (e.g., *Salmonella* spp., *Escherichia coli* O157:H7)	
Water safety threats (e.g., *Vibrio cholerae*, *Cryptosporidium parvum*)	
Category C	
Emerging threat agents (e.g., Nipah virus, hantavirus)	

SUMMARY

- Infectious diseases are spread through contact, droplet, airborne, and vector transmission.
- Common infectious agents include bacteria, viruses, fungi, and parasites.
- The communicability period of a disease depends on the virulence, the number of organisms that are transmitted, the mode of transportation, and the host's resistance.
- If the source of the pandemic is a virulent new pathogen or a mutant form of an older disease, few people will have the antibodies that make them resistant to the disease.
- EMS providers need to be vigilant and report any unexpected influx of patients or other atypical patient trends.

REFERENCES AND ADDITIONAL RESOURCES

Association for Professionals in Infection Control and Epidemiology. (2013). *Guide to infection prevention in emergency medical services*. Washington, DC: Author. Retrieved from https://www.ems.gov/pdf/workforce/Guide_Infection_Prevention_EMS.pdf

Bolyard, E. A., Tablan, O. C., Williams, W. W., Pearson, M. L., Shapiro, C. N., and Deitchman, S. D. (1998). Guideline for infection control in health care personnel, 1998. Hospital Infection Control Practices Advisory Committee. *Infection Control and Hospital Epidemiology, 19*, 407–463. Retrieved from http://id_center.apic.org/Resource_/TinyMceFileManager/Practice_Guidance/IC-HealthCare-Personnel.pdf

Centers for Disease Control and Prevention. (2017, January). National Center for Immunization and Respiratory Diseases (NCIED). Retrieved from https://www.cdc.gov/ncird/index.html

Metropolitan Chicago Healthcare Council. (2012). *Infection prevention and control guidance for EMS providers*. Chicago, IL: Author. Retrieved from http://www.dgprofessionals.com/seavival/INFECTION%20CONTROL%20GUIDANCE%20FOR%20EMS%20PROVIDERS%20CHICAGO%20EMS%202012.pdf

Taubenberger, J. K., and Morens, D. M. (2006). 1918 influenza: The mother of all pandemics. *Emerging Infectious Diseases, 12*(1), 15–22. Retrieved from https://wwwnc.cdc.gov/eid/article/12/1/05-0979_article/

World Health Organization. (n.d.). WHO in emergencies. Retrieved from http://www.who.int/emergencies/en/

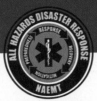

CRITICAL·THINKING SKILL STATION

Mass-Casualty Tabletop Exercise

Exercise Introduction: The purpose of this exercise is improved competencies in response to a multi-casualty incident. The scenario you have responded to is a catering hall with 30 patients with vomiting, nausea, abdominal pain, and cramps.

How will the incident command system be established and utilized?

- If the potential for bioterrorism exists, a unified command between EMS and law enforcement would likely be the most appropriate. If bioterrorism is not suspected, EMS should establish an incident command system.
- The response to this incident will likely not last longer than one operational period, not require supplies beyond those typically available within an EMS system, or incur expenses beyond those typically incurred. As a result, the ICS will not require a planning section chief, logistics sections chief, or finance/administration section chief. A public information officer may be needed if the media presents on the incident scene.

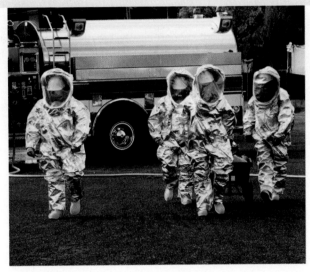

© BenDC/iStock/Getty.

What are the roles of fire and EMS within the response?

- EMS will provide medical care and transportation for the ill patients.
- Once a HAZMAT issue has been reasonably ruled out, there may not be a need for the fire service within the response. However, they may be willing to support EMS with operational tasks, such as staging ambulances and/or tracking patients departing the scene.

What other resources or units may be needed?

- Could this be a criminal event? If the potential exists, law enforcement will be need to be informed.
- Consider involving public health to begin epidemiological investigation. Public health may also be needed to expedite samples being sent for laboratory testing to rule out a bioterrorism agent.

Will an on-scene treatment unit be established?

- The number of transport units and receiving facilities available will influence this decision. An on-scene treatment unit can be utilized to stabilize patients and prepare them for transfer to a receiving facility.

How will patients be transported to tertiary care?

- Patient transport may become more dynamic during a multi-casualty incident. Consider alternative transportation methods such as mass transit buses. Applicable laws and regulations will determine what nontraditional methods of transportation may be acceptable during these events.

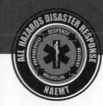

CRITICAL THINKING **SKILL STATION**

Mass-Casualty Tabletop Exercise

How can EMS prepare the receiving facilities for the surge of patients?

- Early notification is critical for receiving facilities to prepare for patient surge. This may be especially true in rural areas and communities with limited receiving facilities.

How should these patients be clinically managed?

- Basic Life Support: support airway, breathing, and circulation.
- Advanced Life Support: IV fluids for dehydration and/or hypotension. Antiemetic medication for symptomatic relief and to maintain patency of the airway.

CHAPTER

7

Active Shooter: Evolving Concepts of Care

OBJECTIVES

After studying this chapter, you will be able to:

- Appreciate the incidence and prevalence of active shooter events in the United States.

- Stay informed regarding the evolving concepts for response to active shooter events.

- List common indications for and limitations to the use of personal protective equipment.

- Gain familiarity with the concept of operating in the warm corridor where specific agency protocols, procedures, and training are allowed.

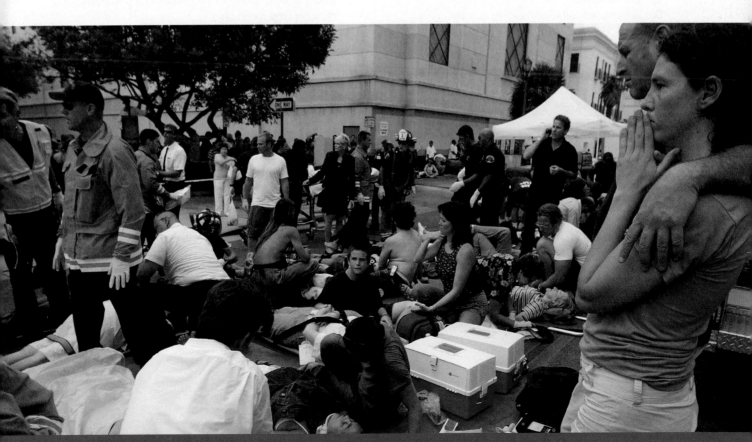

© Carlos Chavez/Los Angeles Times/Getty.

What Is an Active Shooter?

An **active shooter** is an individual actively engaged in killing or attempting to kill people in a confined space or other populated area. In most cases, active shooters use firearms and there is no pattern or method to their selection of victims. Active shooter situations are unpredictable and evolve quickly. Active shooters usually will continue to move throughout a building or area until stopped by law enforcement, suicide, or other intervention. Typically, the deployment of law enforcement is required to stop the shooting and to prevent further harm to victims.

The "active" aspect of the definition implies that both law enforcement personnel and citizens can affect the outcome of the event through their responses. The persistence of these incidents supports the paramount need for training and exercises for law enforcement, other first responders, and citizens alike.

 CHECK YOUR KNOWLEDGE

Active shooter situations:

A. involve shooting for more than 15 minutes.
B. generate more fatalities than wounded patients.
C. are ritualistic.
D. are unpredictable and evolve quickly.

Incidence and Prevalence of Active Shooter Events

The Federal Bureau of Investigation (FBI) has studied active shooter incidents. A study of 160 active shooter incidents between the years 2000 and 2013 provides a perspective on the issue, with an increasing trend of annual incidents (**FIGURE 7-1**).

Incidence

Study of active shooter incidents from 2000 to 2013 reveals the following data:

- An average of 11.4 incidents occurred annually.
- An average of 6.4 incidents occurred in the first 7 years studied, and an average of 16.4 incidents occurred in the last 7 years.
- Seventy percent of the incidents occurred in either a commerce or a business or an educational environment.

active shooter An individual actively engaged in killing or attempting to kill people in a confined space or other populated area.

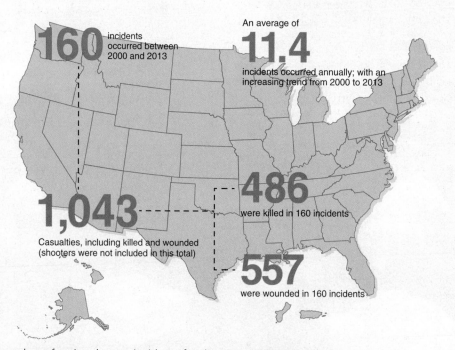

Figure 7-1 Snapshot of active shooter incidents for the years 2000–2013.

Data from Blair, J. Pete, and Schweit, Katherine W. (2014). A Study of Active Shooter Incidents, 2000-2013. Texas State University and Federal Bureau of Investigation Accessed January 25, 2017 from https://www.fbi.gov/file-repository/active-shooter-study-2000-2013-1.pdf.

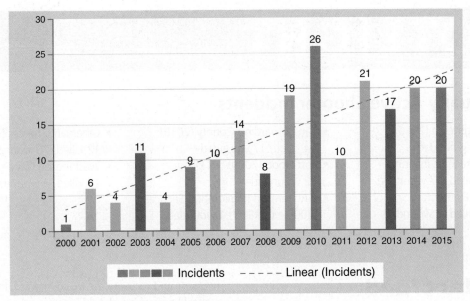

Figure 7-2 Active shooter events for the years 2000–2015.

Data from Schweit, Katherine W. (2016). Active Shooter Incidents in the United States in 2014 and 2015. Washington DC: Federal Bureau of Investigation, U.S. Department of Justice. Accessed January 25, 2017 from https://www.fbi.gov/file-repository/activeshooterincidentsus_2014-2015.pdf ; Blair, J. Pete, and Schweit, Katherine W. (2014). A Study of Active Shooter Incidents, 2000-2013. Texas State University and Federal Bureau of Investigation Accessed January 25, 2017 from https://www.fbi.gov/file-repository/active-shooter-study-2000-2013-1.pdf

- Shootings occurred in 40 of 50 states and the District of Columbia.
- Sixty percent of the incidents ended before police arrived.

Casualties

Casualty statistics relating to the 160 active shooter events between the years 2000 and 2013 include the following:

- Casualties (victims killed and wounded) totaled 1,043. The individual shooters are not included in this total.
- A total of 486 individuals were killed.
- A total of 557 individuals were wounded.
- In 64 incidents (40%), the crime would have fallen within the federal definition of **mass killing**— defined as three or more killed.

Shooters

Data on the shooters in the incidents from 2000 to 2013 include the following:

- All but two incidents involved a single shooter.
- In at least nine incidents, the shooter first shot and killed a family member(s) in a residence before moving to a more public location to continue shooting.
- In at least six incidents, the shooters were female.
- In 64 incidents (40%), the shooters committed suicide; 54 shooters did so at the scene of the crime.

- At least five shooters from four incidents remain at large.

The FBI subsequently added to the study, looking at data from 2014 and 2015. They noted that 15 of the 40 (37.5%) incidents meet the criteria cited in the federal definition of a "mass killing"; that is, they involved "three or more killings in a single incident." This finding is consistent with the FBI's previous study of 160 active shooter incidents that found 40% of the incidents fell within the federal definition of a mass killing (**FIGURE 7-2**).

✓ **CHECK YOUR KNOWLEDGE**

In reviewing the active shooter incidents between 2000 and 2013, the FBI noted that _____ of the incidents ended before police arrived.

A. 75%
B. 60%
C. 40%
D. 25%

mass killing An incident in which three or more are killed.

SPOTLIGHT

High-Casualty Active Shooter Incidents

- The Pulse Nightclub (2016): 49 killed, 53 wounded
- Virginia Polytechnic Institute (2007): 32 killed, 17 wounded
- Sandy Hook Elementary School (2012): 27 killed, 2 wounded
- San Bernardino County (2015): 14 killed, 17 wounded
- Fort Hood (2009): 13 killed, 32 wounded
- Binghamton Immigration Services (2009): 13 killed, 4 wounded
- Cinemark Theater (2012): 12 killed, 70 wounded
- Washington Navy Yard (2013): 12 killed, 3 wounded

The Hartford Consensus

In April 2013, just a few months after the active shooter disaster on December 14, 2012, at Sandy Hook Elementary School in Newtown, Connecticut, the Joint Committee to Create a National Policy to Enhance Survivability from Intentional Mass-Casualty and Active Shooter Events was convened by the American College of Surgeons in collaboration with the medical community and representatives from the federal government, the National Security Council, the U.S. military, the FBI, and governmental and nongovernmental emergency medical response organizations, among other participants. The committee was formed under the guidance and leadership of trauma surgeon Lenworth M. Jacobs, Jr., vice president of academic affairs and chief academic officer at Hartford Hospital, and professor of surgery at the University of Connecticut School of Medicine, to create a protocol for national policy to enhance survivability from active shooter and intentional mass-casualty events. The committee's recommendations, called the Hartford Consensus, currently consist of the following four reports:

- Improving Survival from Active Shooter Events: The Hartford Consensus
- Active Shooter and Intentional Mass-Casualty Events: The Hartford Consensus II
- The Hartford Consensus III: Implementation of Bleeding Control
- The Hartford Consensus IV: A Call for Increased National Resilience

THREAT Response

The response to shooting events has historically involved a segmented, sequential public safety operation first focused on law enforcement goals (stop the shooting), followed by the remainder of the incident, which is typically focused on

response and recovery. As we go forward, initial actions to control hemorrhage should be part of the law enforcement response, and knowledge of hemorrhage control needs to be a core law enforcement skill. Maximizing survival requires an updated and integrated system that can achieve multiple objectives simultaneously.

Recognizing that active shooter incidents can occur in any community, the Hartford Consensus encourages the use of existing emergency medical techniques and equipment, validated by over a decade of well-documented clinical evidence. The Hartford Consensus recommends that an integrated active shooter response should include the critical actions contained in the acronym THREAT:

- **T**hreat suppression
- **H**emorrhage control
- **R**apid **E**xtrication to safety
- **A**ssessment by medical providers
- **T**ransport to definitive care

Life-threatening bleeding from extremity wounds is best controlled initially through use of tourniquets, while internal bleeding resulting from penetrating wounds to the chest and trunk is best addressed through expeditious transport to a hospital setting. THREAT incorporates the proven concepts of self-care and buddy-care.

 CHECK YOUR KNOWLEDGE

The "H" in the Hartford Consensus THREAT acronym means:

A. highly trained intervention teams.
B. hypertonic fluid resuscitation.
C. hybrid EMS and law enforcement deployment.
D. hemorrhage control.

The Hartford Consensus Zones

Response to an active shooter incident applies the same hot, warm, and cold zones as those used in radiation/hazardous materials incident operations (**FIGURE 7-3**). The active shooter hot zone is an area where there is a known hazard or a direct and immediate life-threatening situation—that is, any uncontrolled area where an active shooter could directly engage a rescue team. Within the hot zone, the only care provided is to stop life-threatening external hemorrhage, if tactically feasible, by using a tourniquet.

The active shooter warm zone is an area of indirect threat—that is, an area where law enforcement officials have either cleared or isolated the threat to a level of minimal or mitigated risk. Responders will provide a dedicated patient assessment and initiate appropriate lifesaving interventions if needed. The cold zone in an active shooter event is similar to the treatment area in a mass-casualty event. Due to the dynamic nature of active shooter events, there are no threat-free areas until the threat is neutralized.

 CHECK YOUR KNOWLEDGE

A patient with a pneumothorax and significant trouble breathing will receive a chest decompression in the:

A. hot zone.
B. warm zone.
C. cold zone.
D. treatment sector.

THREAT

The Hartford Consensus
Improving Survival from Active Shooter and Intentional Mass Casualty Events

Hot Zone	**Danger**	Threat Suppression
Warm Zone	**Not Secure**	Hemorrhage Control / Rapid Extrication
Cold Zone	**Safe**	Assess Patient / Transport to Hospital

Figure 7-3 Hartford Consensus zones.

Reproduced from American College of Surgeons (2015 September) "Strategies to Enhance Survival and Intentional Mass Casualty Events." ACS Bulletin Supplements. Chicago: American College of Surgeons. Accessed January 25, 2017 from https://www.facs.org/~/media/files/publications/bulletin/hartford%20 consensus%20compendium.ashx

Personal Protection of the EMS Provider During Active Shooter Incidents

EMS providers responding to active shooter events will be operating in an environment that involves different tactics, techniques, and procedures. This response includes the use of ballistic vests, better situational awareness, and application of concealment and cover concepts. There are important military and law enforcement concepts that the EMS provider should understand:

- **Force protection.** Actions taken by law enforcement to prevent or mitigate hostile actions against personnel, resources, facilities, and critical infrastructures. These actions conserve the operational ability of emergency responders.
- **Concealment.** An object that hides a responder from active shooter observation. It can be natural or human-made. Concealment does not protect from gunfire.
- **Cover.** An object that provides protection from bullets, fragments of exploding rounds, flame, nuclear effects, and biologic and chemical agents. Natural cover includes such objects as logs, trees, stumps, ravines, or hollows. Human-made cover includes vehicles, trenches, walls, rubble, and craters.

active shooter hot zone An area where there is a known hazard or a direct and immediate life-threatening situation (i.e., any uncontrolled area where an active shooter could directly engage a rescue team).

active shooter warm zone An area of indirect threat (i.e., an area where law enforcement officials have either cleared or isolated the threat to a level of minimal or mitigated risk). This area can be considered clear but not secure.

force protection Actions taken by law enforcement to prevent or mitigate hostile actions against personnel, resources, facilities, and critical infrastructures.

concealment An object that hides a responder from active shooter observation.

cover An object that provides protection from bullets, fragments of exploding rounds, flame, nuclear effects, and biologic and chemical agents.

CHECK YOUR KNOWLEDGE

Protection from bullets require that a responder use:

A. cover.
B. camouflage.
C. concealment.
D. countertactics.

Ballistic Vests

There are five types of ballistic vests based on National Institute of Justice (NIJ) body armor standards. The body armor standards, ordered by the level of protection, are presented in the following list. Type IIA vests, for example, provide protection against Type II and Type IIA threats, whereas Type III vests provide protection for Type IIA, Type II, and Type IIIA threats.

1. Type IIA protects against 9-mm and .40-caliber Smith and Wesson bullets.
2. Type II protects against 9-mm and .357-caliber Magnum bullets.
3. Type IIIA protects against .357 SIG and .44-caliber Magnum bullets.
4. Type III protects against rifles, as tested with 7.62-mm full metal jacket (FMJ) bullets.
5. Type IV protects against armor piercing (AP) rifles, as tested with .30-caliber AP bullets.

Statistics from the Bulletproof Vest Partnership/Body Armor Safety Initiative indicate that the majority of vests used by first responders are Type II and Type IIIA.

Ballistic vests are manufactured so that the projectile's kinetic energy is trapped and the energy is disbursed throughout a bigger surface, which ensures it does not pierce the body and damage vital organs. The wearer will still feel the blunt force trauma from the bullet, however.

CHECK YOUR KNOWLEDGE

Emergency service responders tend to use _____ ballistic vests.

A. Type IV and Type IIA
B. Type III and Type IV
C. Type IIIA and Type II
D. Type IV and Type V

Shock Management

Civilian active shooter scenarios present similar injuries and conditions to those seen in combat (in decreasing order of mortality): extremity hemorrhage, tension pneumothorax, and airway obstruction. Each of these wounds is readily treatable with minimal supplies, but they are very time sensitive, and delay in treatment increases the risk of mortality. Because victims in an active shooter incident are more likely to suffer exsanguinating extremity wounds than airway injury, and because a person can bleed to death from a large arterial wound in 2 to 3 minutes while it may take 4 to 5 minutes to die from a compromised airway, the Committee for Tactical Emergency Casualty Care (C-TECC) guidelines place control of external hemorrhage ahead of airway control—replacing the traditional ABC mnemonic (for airway, breathing, circulation) with MARCH (Massive hemorrhage control/Airway support/Respiratory threats/Circulation [prevent shock]/Hypothermia).

Hemorrhage Control

A comprehensive study of U.S. combat fatalities from 2001 to 2011 noted that the incidence of treatable exsanguination deaths related to extremity hemorrhage dropped from 7.8% in a previous study to 2.6% by 2011—a decrease attributed to the implementation of tourniquet use by U.S. forces. To be most effective, the tourniquet must be applied before the victim has lost enough blood to suffer hemorrhagic shock. Despite previous warnings about limb ischemia, there was no preventable loss of limbs resulting from tourniquet ischemia in a case study of 232 patients with tourniquets on 309 extremities.

Anatomic areas such as the neck, groin, and axilla contain large vascular structures and are not amenable to tourniquet placement. Studies at military medical research laboratories have evaluated the efficacy of hemostatic agents and found an advantage in the use of packing hemostatic gauze versus granulated hemostatics. Junctional hemorrhage control devices, such as the Combat Ready Clamp, the Abdominal Aortic Tourniquet, and the Junctional Emergency Treatment Tool, may also be used to control hemorrhage from the groin area (**FIGURE 7-4**).

CHECK YOUR KNOWLEDGE

The first clinical concern when reaching a victim of an active shooter event is:

A. hypothermia.
B. shock.
C. massive hemorrhage.
D. respiratory insult.

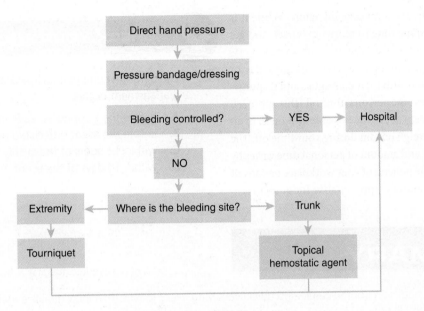

Figure 7-4 Prehospital external hemorrhage control protocol.
© Jones & Bartlett Learning.

Postincident

There are seven major components of critical incident stress management (CISM). The first component of CISM is pre-crisis preparation, which involves stress management education and crisis mitigation training for individuals and organizations. The second component involves post-crisis disaster services, involving school and community support programs. The third component of CISM is defusing, a three-phase, structured, small group discussion that occurs within 12 hours of a crisis. The purpose of defusing is assessment, triage, and acute symptom mitigation. The fourth component is critical incident stress debriefing (CISD), a multiphase, structured group discussion performed 1 to 10 days post-crisis. The purpose of CISD is to mitigate acute symptoms, assess the need for follow-up treatment, and, if possible, provide a sense of post-crisis psychological closure. The fifth component of CISM is one-on-one crisis intervention and counseling throughout the crisis. The sixth component is family crisis intervention and organizational consultation. The seventh and final component of CISM is follow-up treatment and referrals.

Signs of EMS Provider Stress

Signs that an EMS provider is experiencing excessive stress include the following:

- **Bodily sensations and physical effects.** Rapid heart rate, palpitations, muscle tension, headaches, tremors, gastrointestinal distress, nausea, inability to relax when off duty, trouble falling asleep or staying asleep, nightmares, or flashbacks.

- **Strong negative feelings.** Fear or terror in life-threatening situations or perceived danger, anger, frustration, argumentativeness, irritability, deep sadness, and difficulty maintaining emotional balance.
- **Difficulty thinking clearly.** Disorientation or confusion, difficulty problem-solving and making decisions, difficulty remembering instructions, inability to see situations clearly, and distortion and misinterpretation of comments and events.
- **Problematic or risky behaviors.** Unnecessary risk-taking, failure to use personal protective equipment, refusal to follow orders or leave the scene, endangerment of team members, or increased use or misuse of prescription drugs or alcohol.
- **Social conflicts.** Irritability, anger and hostility, blaming, reduced ability to support teammates, conflicts with peers or family, withdrawal, and isolation.

defusing A three-phase, structured, small group discussion that occurs within 12 hours of a crisis as part of critical incident stress management.

critical incident stress debriefing (CISD) A multiphase, structured group discussion performed 1 to 10 days post-crisis as part of critical incident stress management.

Responder resilience is an ongoing effort. While it is a good idea to take some time to reorient yourself and get sufficient sleep after an active shooter event, some experts suggest that responders first go back to work for a day or two to get reacquainted with their colleagues and responsibilities, and then take some personal time off. This approach may help relieve anxiety about the possible aftermath of an event so it does not weigh on you during your time off. The scheduling flexibility and amount of personal time varies by employer, so check the policies of your workplace or consult with your human resources representative for guidance.

CHECK YOUR KNOWLEDGE

The defusing component of critical incident stress management occurs:

A. before the responders leave the incident.
B. before the event is declared over.
C. within 12 hours of the event.
D. within 10 days of the event.

SUMMARY

- An active shooting is an unpredictable and quickly evolving event in which an individual is engaged in killing or attempting to kill people in a confined space or other populated area.
- The Hartford Consensus THREAT acronym helps prioritize response efforts during an active shooter incident. It stands for (1) **T**hreat suppression, (2) **H**emorrhage control, (3) **R**apid **E**xtrication to safety, (4) **A**ssessment by medical providers, and (5) **T**ransport to definitive care.
- Hemorrhage control is the primary prehospital care priority in active shooter events.

REFERENCES AND ADDITIONAL RESOURCES

American College of Surgeons. (2015, September). Strategies to enhance survival in active shooter and intentional mass casualty events: A compendium. *Bulletin, 100*(15). Retrieved from https://www.facs.org/~/media/files/publications/bulletin/hartford%20consensus%20compendium.ashx

Blair, J. P., and Schweit, K. W. (2014). *A study of active shooter incidents, 2000–2013*. Texas State University and Federal Bureau of Investigation, U.S. Department of Justice. Retrieved from https://www.fbi.gov/file-repository/active-shooter-study-2000-2013-1.pdf

Emergency Management Institute. (2015). *IS-907: Active shooter; What you can do. Student manual*. Washington, DC: National Protection and Programs Directorate/Office of Infrastructure Protection, U.S. Department of Homeland Security. Retrieved from https://training.fema.gov/is/courseoverview.aspx?code=IS-907

National Institute of Justice. (2014, December). *Selection and application guide to ballistic-resistant body armor for law enforcement, corrections and public safety*. Washington, DC: U.S. Department of Justice. Retrieved from https://www.ncjrs.gov/pdffiles1/nij/247281.pdf

Office of Health Affairs. (2015, June). *First responder guide for improving survivability in improvised explosive device and/or active shooter incidents*. Washington, DC: U.S. Department of Homeland Security. Retrieved from https://www.dhs.gov/sites/default/files/publications/First%20Responder%20Guidance%20June%202015%20FINAL%202.pdf

Schweit, K. W. (2016). *Active shooter incidents in the United States in 2014 and 2015*. Washington, DC: Federal Bureau of Investigation, U.S. Department of Justice. Retrieved from https://www.fbi.gov/file-repository/activeshooterincidentsus_2014-2015.pdf

Smith, E. R., Jr., and Delaney, J. B. (2013, December). A new response: Supporting paradigm change in EMS' operational medical response to active shooter events. *Journal of Emergency Medical Services*. Retrieved from http://www.c-tecc.org/images/content/Smith.Delaney.Active_ShooterDec2013.pdf

U.S. Department of Homeland Security. (2015). *Active shooter: How to respond*. Retrieved from https://www .dhs.gov/sites/default/files/publications/active-shooter-how-to-respond-508.pdf

U.S. Fire Administration. (2012, June). *Operational templates and guidance for EMS mass incident deployment*. Washington, DC: Federal Emergency Management Administration. Retrieved from https://www.usfa.fema .gov/downloads/pdf/publications/templates_guidance_ems_mass_incident_deployment.pdf

U.S. Fire Administration. (2013, September). *Fire/emergency medical services department operationa l considerations and guide for active shooter and mass casualty incidents*. Washington, DC: Federal Emergency Management Administration. Retrieved from https://www.usfa.fema.gov/downloads/pdf /publications/active_shooter_guide.pdf

Woods, G. L. (2007). Post traumatic stress symptoms and critical stress debriefing (CISD) in emergency medical services (EMS) personnel (Master's thesis). Available from East Tennessee University, Electronic Theses and Dissertations, Paper 2035. Retrieved from http://dc.etsu.edu/etd/2035

CRITICAL THINKING SKILL STATION

All Hazards Disaster Response Active Shooter Tabletop Exercise

Situation Manual—Participant

Exercise Overview

Exercise Name	*All Hazards Disaster Response* Active Shooter Tabletop Exercise
Scope	This exercise is a tabletop, planned for 60 minutes. Exercise play is limited to a facilitated discussion among course participants.
Mission Area(s)	Response
Core Capabilities	Operational coordination Public information and warning Environmental response/health and safety Fatality management services On-scene security, protection, and law enforcement Operational communications Public health, health care, and emergency medical services (EMS) Situational assessment
Objectives	Identify the situation, report critical information, and establish or integrate with an incident command system (ICS). Direct the operations of EMS personnel during the response. Ensure the safety of self and other EMS providers. Interact with the media and the incident public information officer (PIO). Identify proper transportation and disposition of victims.
Threat or Hazard	Active shooter
Scenario	An active shooter event has occurred at a local shopping center. There are numerous patients, and you have been asked to serve as the EMS group leader.
Sponsor	National Association of Emergency Medical Technicians (NAEMT)
Point of Contact	The authors of the *All Hazards Disaster Response (AHDR)* course can be reached at AHDR@lists.naemt.org.

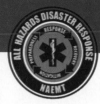

CRITICAL THINKING SKILL STATION

All Hazards Disaster Response Active Shooter Tabletop Exercise

General Information

Exercise Objectives and Core Capabilities

Table 1 describes the expected outcomes for the exercise. The objectives are linked to core capabilities, which are distinct critical elements necessary to achieve the specific mission area(s).

TABLE 1 Exercise Objectives and Associated Core Capabilities

Exercise Objective	Core Capability
Identify the situation, report critical information, and establish or integrate with an ICS.	Operational coordination On-scene security, protection, and law enforcement Operational communications Public health, health care, and EMS Situational assessment
Direct the operations of EMS personnel during the response.	Operational coordination Operational communications Public health, health care, and EMS
Ensure the safety of self and other EMS providers.	Environmental response/health and safety
Interact with the media and the incident PIO.	Public information and warning
Identify proper transportation and disposition of victims.	Operational coordination Public health, health care, and EMS Fatality management services

Participant Roles and Responsibilities

The term *participant* encompasses many groups of people, not just those playing in the exercise. Groups of participants involved in the exercise, and their respective roles and responsibilities, are as follows:

- **Players.** Players are personnel who have an active role in discussing or performing their regular roles and responsibilities during the exercise. Players discuss or initiate actions in response to the simulated emergency. The role of players is performed by AHDR course participants.
- **Facilitators.** Facilitators provide situation updates and moderate discussions. They also provide additional information or resolve questions as required. Key exercise planning team members also may assist as subject-matter experts during the exercise. The role of facilitator(s) is performed by AHDR course faculty.

Exercise Structure

This exercise will be a multimedia-facilitated exercise. Players will participate in the following two modules:

- Module 1: Background and Initial Response
- Module 2: EMS Group Leader

CRITICAL THINKING SKILL STATION

All Hazards Disaster Response Active Shooter Tabletop Exercise

Each module begins with an update that summarizes key events occurring within that period. After the updates, participants review the situation and engage in group discussions of appropriate response issues.

After these group discussions, participants will engage in a moderated plenary discussion in which a spokesperson from each group presents a synopsis of the group's actions, based on the scenario. The AHDR course faculty will facilitate the plenary discussion.

Exercise Guidelines

- This exercise will be held in an open, low-stress, no-fault environment. Varying viewpoints, even disagreements, are expected.
- Respond to the scenario using your knowledge of current plans and capabilities (i.e., you may use only existing assets) and insights derived from your training.
- Decisions are not precedent setting and may not reflect your organization's final position on a given issue. This exercise is an opportunity to discuss and present multiple options and possible solutions.
- Issue identification is not as valuable as suggestions and recommended actions that could improve response efforts. Problem-solving efforts should be the focus.

Exercise Assumptions and Artificialities

In any exercise, assumptions and artificialities may be necessary to complete play in the time allotted and/or account for logistical limitations. Exercise participants should accept that assumptions and artificialities are inherent in any exercise and should not allow these considerations to negatively impact their participation. During this exercise, the following conditions apply:

- The exercise is conducted in a no-fault learning environment.
- The exercise scenario is plausible, and events occur as they are presented.
- All players receive information at the same time.

Module 1: Background and Initial Response

You are a mid-level supervisor in a small, rural community. You are employed by a progressive private ambulance company that is part of a contemporary EMS system.

Under the county medical director, county fire chief, and county sheriff, all allied resources and personnel undergo quarterly, all-risk first responder training. In this system, all first responders are trained to the hazardous materials First Responder Operational (FRO) level, and all have been trained in Prehospital Trauma Life Support and National Incident Management System ICS-100 and ICS-200.

Additionally, your system has an automatic aid system agreement and deploys resources using global positioning system (GPS) technology that enables automatic vehicle locating (AVL). Lastly, all fire, EMS, and police radio frequencies are programmed into each other's radios and the radios are encrypted.

Although you work for a small, private agency, all resources are well trained and present a multitude of assets at your disposal. Many outside, allied resources can be on scene in your town within 7 to 10 minutes.

You are dispatched for a report of shots fired at a local shopping center. Initial dispatch reports indicate there may be as many as 15 victims and the shooter may still be present.

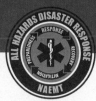

CRITICAL THINKING SKILL STATION

All Hazards Disaster Response Active Shooter Tabletop Exercise

Questions

Discuss the issues raised in the Module 1 scenario. Identify any critical issues, decisions, requirements, or questions that should be addressed.

The following questions are provided as suggested subjects that you may wish to address as the discussion progresses. These questions are not a definitive list of concerns to be addressed, nor is there a requirement to address every question.

1. What are your initial considerations as you approach the scene?
2. What considerations will your initial scene size-up include?
3. What secondary hazards may be present?
4. How will you establish incident command if you are first on scene?
5. How will you integrate with the ICS if it has already been established?
6. When would you enter the facility to care for patients?
7. What types of clinical injury patterns would you expect to see, and how would they be treated?
8. As you are arriving on scene, a woman and a man carrying a video camera approach you, saying they are with the local news. What should you do?

Module 2: EMS Group Leader

Law enforcement entered the building and engaged the shooter, who then committed suicide, prior to your arrival. The first arriving ambulance crew made entry to the building with law enforcement and has performed START triage. There are 14 victims: 4 tagged red, 7 yellow, and 3 black. You currently have three ambulances in your staging area, and the first arriving ambulance crew began setting up a treatment area after finishing with triage. The incident commander and operations section chief ask you to serve as the EMS group leader.

Questions

Discuss the issues raised in the Module 2 scenario. Identify any critical issues, decisions, requirements, or questions that should be addressed.

The following questions are provided as suggested subjects that you may wish to address as the discussion progresses. These questions are not a definitive list of concerns to be addressed, nor is there a requirement to address every question.

1. What is your role as the EMS group leader?
2. What information should regularly be communicated and to whom?
3. If there is a conflict with a law enforcement officer on the scene, who would you address this with?
4. How will patients be prepared for transport?
5. What would you do if an EMS provider within your group were injured during the operation?
6. The PIO for the event has approached you to get information about victims to answer media inquiries. What information can you provide?
7. Once all live patients have been transported from the scene, EMS personnel are asking if they should transport the deceased individuals. What should you tell them?

GLOSSARY

active shooter An individual actively engaged in killing or attempting to kill people in a confined space or other populated area.

active shooter hot zone An area where there is a known hazard or a direct and immediate life-threatening situation (i.e., any uncontrolled area where an active shooter could directly engage a rescue team).

active shooter warm zone An area of indirect threat (i.e., an area where law enforcement officials have either cleared or isolated the threat to a level of minimal or mitigated risk). This area can be considered clear but not secure.

acute radiation syndrome A serious illness that can result from exposure to very high levels of radiation, usually over a short period. The amount of radiation that a person's body absorbs is called the radiation dose.

alpha particle A particle with two neutrons and two protons that is ejected from the nucleus of a radioactive atom. The particle is identical to the nucleus of a helium atom.

ambulance strike team An ICS resource consisting of five ambulances and a supervisor or support vehicle operating under a shared communication system.

asymptomatic carrier An infected patient who has no knowledge of the infection but is capable of transmitting the disease to others.

beta particle A high-energy, high-speed electron emitted from the nucleus of a radioactive atom and most frequently found in nuclear fallout. Because this electron is from the nucleus of the atom, it is called a beta particle to distinguish it from the electrons that orbit the atom.

biologic agent A pathogen or toxin that may be used as a weapon to spread disease or cause injury to humans.

CBRN Abbreviation for the constellation of chemical, biologic, radiologic, and nuclear hazards.

chronic radiation dose A dose of ionizing radiation received either continuously or intermittently over a prolonged period.

communicable disease Any infectious disease transmitted from one person or animal to another.

concealment An object that hides a responder from active shooter observation.

consensus formula A formula used to calculate a range for resuscitative-phase fluid replacement (lactated Ringer's solution) in the first 24 hours when the fluid shifts and the risk for hypovolemic shock is the greatest.

cover An object that provides protection from bullets, fragments of exploding rounds, flame, nuclear effects, and biologic and chemical agents.

critical incident stress debriefing (CISD) A multiphase, structured group discussion performed 1 to 10 days post-crisis as part of critical incident stress management.

defusing A three-phase, structured, small group discussion that occurs within 12 hours of a crisis as part of critical incident stress management.

disaster A sudden, calamitous event that seriously disrupts the functioning of a community or society and causes human, material, and economic or environmental losses that exceed the community's or society's ability to cope using its own resources.

division A supervisory level established to divide an incident into geographic areas of operations.

dose The amount of radiation energy deposited or absorbed in the body.

dose rate A measurement of how fast the radiation energy is deposited; also known as rate of exposure.

epidemic A disease outbreak in which many people in a community or region become infected with the same disease.

evacuation The rapid movement of people away from the immediate threat or impact of a disaster to a safer place of shelter.

evacuation warning The alert issued to people in an affected area of a potential threat to life and property.

force protection Actions taken by law enforcement to prevent or mitigate hostile actions against personnel, resources, facilities, and critical infrastructures.

gamma radiation Penetrating electromagnetic radiation of a kind arising from the radioactive decay of atomic nuclei.

gray (Gy) A unit used to measure whole-body exposure to ionizing radiation. 1 Gy = 100 rad.

group A supervisory level established to divide the incident into functional areas of operations.

immediate evacuation order An order requiring the immediate movement of people out of an affected area due to an imminent threat to life.

immediately dangerous to life and health (IDLH) Defined by the U.S. National Institute for Occupational Safety and Health as exposure to airborne contaminants that is "likely to cause death or immediate or delayed permanent adverse health effects or prevent escape from such an environment."

impact phase The occurrence of an actual event, such as a hurricane or mass-casualty incident.

improvised nuclear device (IND) An illicit nuclear weapon bought, stolen, or otherwise originating from a nuclear state, or a weapon fabricated by a terrorist group from illegally obtained fissile nuclear weapons material that produces a nuclear explosion.

incident action plan (IAP) A continuously updated outline of the overall strategy, tactics, and risk management plans developed by the incident commander.

incident command system (ICS) An emergency response system that defines the roles and responsibilities to be assumed by personnel and the operating procedures to be used in the management and direction of emergency operations.

incident commander (IC) The person responsible for all aspects of a response to an incident, including developing incident objectives, managing all incident operations, setting priorities, and defining the incident command system for the specific response; the IC position must always be filled.

infectious disease An illness caused by pathogenic organisms such as bacteria, viruses, fungi, and parasites. Most infectious diseases, such as the common cold, are not life threatening.

mass-casualty incident (MCI) Any incident in which emergency medical services resources, such as personnel and equipment, are overwhelmed by the number and severity of casualties.

mass killing An incident in which three or more are killed.

National Incident Management System (NIMS) A plan that provides a consistent nationwide template to enable federal, state, tribal, and local governments; the private sector; and nongovernmental organizations to work together to prepare for, prevent, respond to, recover from, and mitigate the effects of incidents, regardless of cause, size, location, or complexity, so as to reduce the loss of life, damage to property, and harm to the environment.

neutron radiation A kind of ionizing radiation that consists of free neutrons. Free neutrons are released from atoms as a result of nuclear fission or nuclear fusion and then react with nuclei of other atoms to form new isotopes, which, in turn, may produce radiation.

pandemic An epidemic that sweeps the planet, reaching all seven continents.

patient exit point (PEP) The physical location through which the patient exits the scene via the transport unit (air or ground); it is here that the transport stub is collected (by the transport recorder) from the disaster tag and affixed to the transport record. If available, the departure should be scanned into the patient tracking system.

patient intake point (PIP) The physical location prior to entering the treatment areas through which all patients are funneled and where a disaster tag is applied. When possible, the disaster tag should be scanned into the patient tracking system.

primary triage The process by which initial prehospital providers assess the scope of the incident, including the number of casualties, the severity of their condition, and the additional or specialized resources needed.

prodrome phase Preparation for a specific event that has been identified as inevitable, such as an incoming hurricane or an imminent failure of an element of the infrastructure.

quiescence phase The time in between disasters or mass-casualty incidents during which risk assessment and mitigation activities should be performed.

radiation sickness Damage to the body caused by a large dose of radiation often received over a short period (acute). The amount of radiation absorbed by the body—the absorbed dose—determines how sick the patient will be.

radiologic dispersal device (RDD) A conventional explosive device with radiologic contaminants present, or any device that can disperse radioactive material.

radiologic exposure device (RED) A simple radiologic device designed to expose people to radiation.

radiologic incendiary device (RID) A radiologic device pairing fire with radioactive contamination.

recovery and reconstruction phase Use of community resources to endure, emerge from, and rebuild after the effects of a disaster.

response phase The emergency services rescue and relief operations to save lives and preserve communities after the impact of an event.

secondary triage A more detailed assessment performed when the patient arrives at the treatment/transport area.

shelter-in-place Selecting a small, interior room, with no or few windows, and taking refuge there.

sievert (Sv) A unit of dose equivalent (the biologic effect of ionizing radiation), equal to an effective dose of a joule of energy per kilogram of recipient mass. 1 Sv = 100 rem.

sort, assess, lifesaving interventions, treatment/triage (SALT) A triage system that is a national guideline for handling MCIs.

special needs population Groups whose needs are not fully addressed by traditional service providers or who feel they cannot comfortably or safely access and use the standard resources offered in disaster preparedness, relief, and recovery.

strategic level The command level that entails the overall direction and goals of the incident.

surge capacity The ability to evaluate and care for a markedly increased volume of patients that challenges or exceeds normal operating capacity.

tactical level The command level in which objectives must be achieved to meet the strategic goals. The tactical-level supervisor or officer is responsible for completing assigned objectives.

task level The command level in which specific tasks are assigned to units or teams; these tasks are geared toward meeting tactical-level requirements.

virulence The power of a microorganism to produce disease.

weapon of mass destruction (WMD) A nuclear, biologic, or chemical weapon that can cause a high order of destruction.

worried well People who do not need medical treatment but who seek it for the sake of being reassured.

INDEX

Note: Page numbers followed by *f* and *t* indicate material in figures and tables, respectively.